Oxford Medical Publications

World nutrition and nutrition education

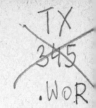

World nutrition and nutrition education

Edited by
H.M. SINCLAIR
AND
G.R. HOWAT

Oxford
OXFORD UNIVERSITY PRESS
New York Toronto
UNESCO, Paris
1980

Oxford University Press, Walton Street, Oxford OX2 6DP

OXFORD LONDON GLASGOW
NEW YORK TORONTO MELBOURNE WELLINGTON
KUALA LUMPUR SINGAPORE JAKARTA HONG KONG TOKYO
DELHI BOMBAY CALCUTTA MADRAS KARACHI
NAIROBI DAR ES SALAAM CAPE TOWN

First published 1980 by the United Nations Educational,
Scientific and Cultural Organization, 7, Place de Fontenoy,
75700, Paris, France and Oxford University Press, Walton
Street, Oxford OX2 6DP, United Kingdom.

British Library Cataloguing in Publication Data

World nutrition and nutrition education.
(Oxford medical publications).
1. Nutrition — Congresses
I. Sinclair, Hugh Macdonald   II. Howat, G R
III. Unesco   IV. Series
641.1   TX345   79-41326

ISBN 0-19-261176-3 (O.U.P.)

ISBN 92-3-101-736-5 (UNESCO)

Set by Hope Services, Abingdon
Printed in Great Britain
by J. W. Arrowsmith Ltd., Bristol

FRANCIS AYLWARD

1911-78

The Conver er of the Conference on which this book was based was Dr Francis Aylward, Ph.D., D.Sc., Emeritus Professor and former Head of the Department of Food Science at the University of Reading. He had most of the responsibility for the pre-Conference arrangements in the busy months leading up to it and also for all the arrangements during the Conference itself. The success of the Conference was, without doubt, due in very large measure to the care and diligence with which these arrangements were made.

Professor Aylward also gathered together the different papers for publication as he expected to act as Editor of this book. It is with much regret that we have to place on record that he died suddenly in hospital in Reading on 28 September 1978.

The task of acting as Editors of this book therefore fell to us and we would like to express our appreciation of the efficient way in which the earlier work was done by Professor Aylward. It has made our task as Editors much easier than it otherwise would have been.

H.M.S.
G.R.H.

Preface

Although many important conferences have been held throughout the world on different aspects of human nutrition in the past few decades, the Oxford Conference on Nutrition Education held in September 1977 was the first large international gathering devoted specifically to education in human nutrition. This book gives the edited and updated proceedings of the Conference. The fact that the Conference attracted about 330 persons from 67 different countries and five international organizations indicates clearly the awareness in the minds of many people working in the field of human nutrition of the need for attention to be given to the subject.

The wide range of disciplines represented and the variety of interests present meant that the substance of the papers covered a very wide spectrum. Indeed one discussion group reported that in the minds of some members nutrition education appeared to be in the middle of an identity crisis. However it was clear, both from papers submitted and from the discussions which followed them, that nutrition education covers a wide range of educational activities ranging from advanced courses given in universities and other institutions of higher learning to *ad hoc* advice given to anxious parents by overworked health visitors in bush clinics to which ailing children had been brought for treatment. From such a broad basis of interests it was clear that further thinking and discussion are necessary before a full coherent picture about the nature and status of nutrition education emerges.

It was appropriate that the conference was organized by the International Union of Nutrition Societies (IUNS) and by the United Nations Educational, Scientific and Cultural Organization (UNESCO), both of which are actively involved in nutritional matters in many parts of the world. Whatever the exact scope and character of nutrition education there can be no doubt that essentially its aim is to extend the great body of knowledge of nutrition which has been amassed by painstaking research carried out in laboratories and by field studies of different population groups in many countries of the world. Some of this work has produced significant results which are not yet fully utilized by governments and other agencies which have responsibility for ensuring that the populations over which they have responsibility are adequately fed and that malnutrition is avoided. While in the minds of most people malnutrition is associated with low intake of food in developing countries, there is increasing evidence that some industrialized countries have now to contend with the malnutrition of affluence arising from overconsumption of certain types of food.

How nutrition education could best be carried out, to which groups of the population it should be directed, and what educational methodology was most applicable, as well as what information should be passed on, were some of the matters which were dealt with informally as well as in the formal papers given in the different sessions of the Conference.

UNESCO has already a fine record in nutrition education. In 1970 a programme of nutrition education was approved by the Sixteenth Session of the UNESCO General Conference, for 'improving and supporting education in nutrition, health, and home economics'. Since then the UNESCO nutrition education programme has been reconfirmed and developed.

The specific aim of programmes set up by UNESCO is the development of educational instruments to help member states to develop and improve their own programmes in nutrition education, by holding meetings, seminars, training courses, and consultations. In addition, the status of existing nutrition education programmes is assessed to enable future action to be planned accordingly.

UNESCO has been concerned with the identification of local food and nutrition problems and its aims are that nutrition education is included at all levels in educational programmes, and that equal access to education in nutrition is given to boys and young men as well as to girls and young women.

Since UNESCO has moved into this field it has been encouraged to note that Member States, including those in the developing countries, are becoming aware of nutrition problems in relation to education in general and are bringing these problems into discussion at the highest level. For example, the Conference of Ministers of Education of African Member States in Lagos in 1976 noted that health and nutrition education was currently taking place in some African states as one aspect of the effort to make educational systems more relevant, and recommended that the nutrition education programme of UNESCO should be expanded.

Similarly the Asian Programme of Education Innovation for Development (APEID) decided that its nineteen Member States would include better health and nutrition among five priority concerns which innovation in education should contribute to and promote. This support is likely to be very considerable, because the programme is determined and approved by the national authorities themselves and priority areas are defined at the regional level by matching the needs expressed with the resources offered.

IUNS and UNESCO co-operate closely at an international level, with IUNS providing professional advice and generally acting in a consultant capacity to UNESCO.

An address on behalf of the Director-General of UNESCO expressing his best wishes for the success of the Conference was read at the opening session of the Conference. A letter from the Rt. Hon. Judith Hart, MP, then Minister for Overseas Development in the British Government, was also read at the opening session. In expressing her good wishes for the success of the Conference the Minister recalled some of the earlier contributions by the British Government in the field of nutrition in many countries of the Commonwealth. Both these letters are included in full in this book.

During the various sessions of the Conference nutrition education was considered in both formal and non-formal educational patterns. Within the former there is now a recognized place for nutrition education in many countries. Even so such recognition is often slight and is offered only to certain groups of students. At university level, however, there is often a real awareness of the subject. In many universities there are departments dealing with food science and technology in which nutrition education plays an integral part. Some departments include the word 'nutrition' as part of their name, e.g., 'Department of Food Science and Nutrition'.

Similarly, in teacher-training colleges the home economics departments invariably include some nutrition education as part of the course. However, the majority of students in home economics departments are women. Some colleges, however, include nutrition education as part of biology courses and there both men and women students are included. This limitation in the scope of the students to whom the subject is taught was noted in some of the papers read to the Conference and in subsequent discussions.

In schools, both at elementary and secondary level, nutrition education increasingly finds a place in the curriculum. Even so such instruction can be given only when there are trained staff and adequate teaching facilities.

Non-formal nutrition education—and the papers presented show how wide a field this is—is an area which needs much further study if the instruction is to achieve any worthwhile impact. Because of the very limited formal teaching of education in the past it is understandable that among adults there is a great need for better understanding of almost all nutritional matters. This is true not only in the developing countries but also in the industrialized countries.

The malnutrition of affluence arising from over-eating, or at least from eating too much of certain types of foods, is now recognized as a potentially serious matter among the young. This type of malnutrition is shown in obesity, some kinds of heart disease, and dental caries to name a few of the undesirable physical conditions which can be produced. Participants at the conference were, however, aware that a fuller knowledge of nutrition and a widespread education in its principles would not prevent some of these undesirable aspects of malnutrition arising in certain groups of the population. A high consumption of food, like an addiction to tobacco, is not something which is easily discarded.

This book includes most of the papers presented at the plenary sessions, some of the papers presented at the panel discussions, and gives some of the conclusions reached in the discussion groups. When no formal conclusions were reached, the group discussions are summarized.

The papers which were submitted and read in French have been translated by accredited translators into English. To ensure that, as far as possible, a similar form of presentation is maintained throughout the book a few minor editorial changes have been made when this seemed desirable.

H.M.S.
G.R.H.

The views expressed in this volume are those of the editors and of the individual contributors, who represent a wide variety of backgrounds. Hence, their opinions are not necessarily those of UNESCO. Similarly, none of the contributions should be taken as reflecting the position of UNESCO concerning the legal status of the countries or territories mentioned, the authorities governing those countries or territories, or their boundaries and frontiers.

Contents

List of contributors

Dr. S. Amcoff, Department of Educational Research, Uppsala University, Sweden.

Professor F. Aylward (deceased), formerly Emeritus Professor of Food Science, University of Reading, U.K.

Dr. K. Bagchi, Senior Nutrition Officer, Nutrition Unit, World Health Organization, Geneva, Switzerland.

Professor F.L. Bartels, Science Division, UNESCO, Paris, France.

Professor S. Berger, Head of Department of Human Nutrition, Agricultural University of Warsaw, Poland.

Professor M. Cépède, Head of Department of Social and Comparative Agricultural Economics, National Institute of Agronomy, Paris, France.

Professor W.J. Darby, Director, Nutrition Foundation, New York and Professor, Vanderbilt University, Tennessee, U.S.A.

Professor M. Egly, French Agency for Technical Cooperation, Paris, France.

Professor H. Ghassemi, Director, Institute of Nutritional Sciences and Food Technology, Teheran, Iran.

Professor C. Gopalan, Director-General, Indian Council for Medical Research, New Delhi, India.

Dr. G.A. Griffin, Teachers' College, Columbia University, New York, U.S.A.

Dr. G. Guru, Assistant Coordinator of Nutrition Education, Indian Council for Medical Research, New Delhi, India.

Professor H.H. Hansen, Department of Nutrition and Biochemistry, Royal Danish School of Educational Studies, Copenhagen, Denmark.

Dr. M.A. Hamilton, School of Education, University of the West Indies, Kingston, Jamaica.

Dr. E. Hookham, Nutrition Officer, UNESCO, Paris, France.

Professor G.R. Howat, formerly Department of Nutrition, University of Reading, England, and University of Ife, Nigeria.

Dr. S. Icaza, Director, School of Nutrition, University of San Carlos, Guatemala.

Dr. J.M. MacNaughton, Senior Officer, Food Policy and Nutrition Division, FAO, Rome, Italy.

Dr. C. Maxwell, Organisation for Economic Co-operation and Development, Paris.

Dr. F.D.S. Ngegba, Principal and Regional Director, Bunumba Teachers College, Kenema, Sierra Leone.

Dr. M. Park, Programme Officer, UNICEF, Seoul.

Dr. C. Reilly, Food and Nutrition Unit, Oxford Polytechnical College, U.K.

Professor I. Raw, Centre for Biomedical Education, The City College, New York, U.S.A.

Professor H.M. Sinclair, Director, International Institute of Human Nutrition; Visiting Professor of Food Science, University of Reading, U.K.

Dr. L.J. Tepley, Senior Nutritionist, UNICEF, New York, U.S.A.

Ms. B. Trimmer-Smith, UNICEF, New York, U.S.A.

Professor A.S. Truswell, Department of Nutrition, Queen Elizabeth College, University of London, U.K.

Dr. R. Wolf, Teachers' College, Columbia University, New York, U.S.A.

Opening speeches

Address to the Conference by Dr Emmy Hookham, Division of Science, Technical and Vocational Education, UNESCO, representing the Director-General of UNESCO, Amadou-Mahtar M'Bow.

On behalf of the Director-General of UNESCO, I should like to say that it is both a pleasure and an honour to be present at the opening session of the first International Conference on Nutrition Education, organized by the International Union of Nutritional Sciences with support from UNESCO. I wish to convey to you the best wishes of the Director-General for the success of the Conference.

It is also most appropriate that the Conference is taking place at Oxford University, which has contributed so much to the development of research, new knowledge, education, and leadership in the world community.

The role of education in the development of men and women and society has been a crucial one. Different ideologies have stressed different fundamental values in life and the purpose of human existence. Interwoven in this picture are political, social, economic, ethical, religious, and scientific aspects. Emphasis has been placed on one or the other of these aspects in various societies at different periods of development.

Central to the debates of the world community at this midway point in the Second United Nations Development Decade is the establishment of a new economic and social order in which peace will reign, available resources will be preserved, and such crucial problems as poverty, illiteracy, disease, mal- and undernutrition, and inequalities will be eradicated. To every man and woman's right to adequate nutrition could be added the right to be born with the fullest capacity for growth and development.

The impact of mal- and undernutrition on national development has probably never been more strongly and explicitly expressed as by the Director-General of the Swedish International Development Agency (SIDA) Ernst Michanek, at the opening of the Seminar on Nutrition: A Priority in African Development, sponsored by the Dag Hammarskjöld Foundation in 1972:

To attack illiteracy without simultaneously attacking mal- and undernutrition, which reduce learning capacity, seems hopeless, to put it mildly. To develop a general health service without beginning at the beginning, that is to say with the building up of the human body, is simply not economical. To increase food production without preserving the real value in foods currently produced . . . is wasted effort. To invest in employment without at the same time improving potential manpower capacity and without also improving nutritional conditions is unproductive.

The improvement of the world nutrition and food situation requires various types of intervention and education, particularly nutrition education, which is the theme of this Conference, plays a major role and is a major force in a global attack on nutrition and food problems. In this connection, the Director-General of UNESCO, in his address to the 59th session of the Economic Social Council of the United Nations (ECOSOC), said:

Education and communication must contribute to providing people with the knowledge and know-how which will enable them more effectively to combat, by their own efforts, disease, malnutrition and poor living conditions in general. At the same time, education and communication must enable them to become fully aware of their conditions and of the role which, through their own actions, they can play in the transformation of society.

Improvements in the overall living conditions of a people facilitate the acquirement of a better nutritional status, but it is only when a person also knows and understands what constitutes his or her nutritional requirements and their fulfilment for the individual and the family within the context of locally available resources that individual nutritional status improves. In the experience of the most affluent societies of the world there is clear evidence that economic and social improvement does not automatically guarantee improvement of nutritional status. People still need to know how to utilize their food resources.

The role of education in development and the role of nutrition education in the improvement of a country's food and nutrition situation have not hitherto been adequately understood by the policy-makers of the world community in general. An illustration in point is that of the problem of blind children. It has been estimated that the total annual cost of protecting one million children aged between one and five all over the world against the risk of xerophthalmia would be around $ 3 million; but the recognition of what people can do themselves to prevent blindness, even with a minimum of nutritional knowledge and skills and at a minimum cost of a few cents per year, is hardly acknowledged.

It is encouraging, however, that many countries are now setting up national food and nutrition policy and planning bodies to assist policy-makers in making the appropriate decisions regarding nutrition. Nutrition education and education about the food and nutrition situation in a country and in the world is indispensable for public support of a nutrition and food policy and the implications of this policy.

The holding of this first International Conference on the promotion and improvement of nutrition and food education at all levels and in all types of education is therefore very timely. In your deliberations you will discuss major nutritional problems in developed and developing countries as a basis for educational action. Regarding the implementation of nutrition education programmes, which will be the main focus of your discussion, there are several components of importance to consider if educational results are to be achieved. There are the questions of relevance, curriculum design, methodologies and technology, as well as the question of change and change processes.

Central to the implementation, however, is the question of qualified personnel which requires both technical and pedagogical training. Without qualified personnel for the various educational tasks little can be achieved.

In conclusion, the task before you, which involves working out guidelines for the improvement of nutrition education as an effective intervention to improve the nutrition and food situation in the world, is most challenging and important.

I wish you every success in your deliberations.

Text of the message sent to the Conference by the Rt. Hon. Dame Judith Hart, MP, then Minister for Overseas Development in the British Government.

As Minister for Overseas Development and as Chairman of the United Kingdom National Commission for UNESCO, I am glad to have this opportunity to send you a message of welcome to this important conference on Nutrition Education which has been organized by the IUNS.

I am delighted that UNESCO itself and the UK National Commission are among the organizations which have helped to make it possible.

I particularly welcome the fact that some 70 representatives are attending from developing countries; as Minister for Overseas Development the nutritional problems of the developing countries are of deep concern to me. I am sure you will all recall my Ministry's paper on British Aid and the Relief of Malnutrition published in 1975 which was the report of a committee set up to study and advise on the general problems of protein deficiency with special reference to the needs of the poorest countries. My Ministry is trying to increase its capacity for helping to solve such nutritional problems, and this is an integral part of our policy of aid to the poorest.

Two of the main themes in current thinking about nutrition are the need for nutritional surveillance and the need for developing national food and nutrition policies. These two elements are, however, incomplete without a third—the involvement and co-operation of the people. If any policy is to work, people must have a better understanding of their nutritional needs and of the best way to use their resources. Nutrition education aimed at increasing this understanding is therefore very important, but is also very difficult. There are so few examples of successful nutrition education programmes. It is obvious that the type of education needed and the means of delivering it must vary with local circumstances. This is not a subject on which it is possible to export expertise—or only to a very limited extent. The fact that this conference is being held in Oxford in no way implies, I am sure, that any of us in the host country think that we know the answers. The aim, rather is to provide a forum in which people can exchange experience and perhaps establish collaborative programmes.

I understand that the British Council is making arrangements for those who wish, after the conference, to visit UK universities and institutions where work on nutrition is being undertaken. I am sure that these institutions will benefit greatly from such contacts.

I wish you all success in your discussions and look forward to hearing the results.

Section I
The nutritional background

1 The nutrition of the individual

H.M. SINCLAIR

BIOCHEMICAL INDIVIDUALITY

The most distinguished period in Oxford's scientific history was the middle of the seventeenth century when Robert Boyle (1627–91), one of Britain's greatest experimental scientists, settled in the city about the end of 1655. Amongst the distinguished group he gathered around him (and who later formed the Royal Society) was Richard Lower (1631–91), pupil and assistant of the great physician Thomas Willis (1621–75). In February 1665 Lower drew off blood from the jugular vein of a small dog until it was nearly dead, and then introduced blood from the cervical artery of a large dog, repeating the process until the blood of two large dogs had been passed into the small dog which, after the jugular was sewn up, 'jumped down from the table and . . . began to fondle its master and roll on the grass to clean itself of blood.' The following year Robert Boyle wrote to Lower for details of this experiment to be communicated to the Royal Society. When a group that included the diarist Samuel Pepys (1633–1703) discussed a repetition of the experiment, 'This did give occasion to many pretty wishes, as of the blood of a Quaker to be let into an Archbishop.' Lower, however, saw blood transfusion as a means of improving health, and in 1667 supervised the transfusion of sheep's blood into a Cambridge bachelor of divinity who was considered unduly extrovert. Despite being paid 20 s., he ran away when Lower tried to repeat the experiment for the benefit of his mental condition. It was quickly found that transfusion was usually followed by dark urine, pain in the region of the kidney, rapid pulse, prostration, and death. The cause was unknown until Landsteiner (1868–1943) (1900) discovered the major blood groups and showed that serious reactions occurred when antibodies present in the plasma of the recipient agglutinated the donor's red cells. These erythrocyte antigens are now numbered in hundreds.

Two years after Landsteiner's paper, *The Lancet* published one by Dr A.E. Garrod (1857–1936) entitled 'The incidence of alcaptonuria: a study in chemical individuality' (Garrod 1902). This paper for the first time established that human beings had biochemical differences that were often genetically determined; he concluded 'that just as no two individuals of a species are absolutely identical in bodily structure neither are their chemical processes carried out on exactly the same lines.' His paper recognized for the first time an example of Mendelian recessive inheritance in man. Garrod summarized his studies in his classic Croonian Lectures of 1908, and in his monograph *Inborn errors of metabolism* in 1909 which was revised in 1923. Three fortunate attributes allowed Garrod to make one of the greatest generalizations in medical science: he was a paediatrician, and therefore noticed that the disorders he studied often resulted from consanguineous marriages, and whereas one or more sibs were involved the parents were usually normal; he was a biochemist, friend of Hopkins (1861–1947) (to whom he dedicated his second edition in 1923), and son of a great biochemist (Sir Alfred Garrod (1819–1907) who made what has been described as the first quantitative biochemical investigation on living man when he established the increased blood uric acid in patients with gout); he was a friend of Bateson (1861–1926), the great Cambridge geneticist at the time when Mendel's work was rediscovered. Discussing the control of metabolic reactions by specific enzymes, Garrod wrote as early as 1909: 'If any one step in the process fail the intermediate product in being at the point of arrest will escape further change, just as when the film of a biograph is brought to a standstill the moving figures are left foot in air.' When in 1958 Beadle received a Nobel Prize for his part in the 'discovery that genes act by regulating definite chemical events' (one gene, one enzyme), he paid eloquent tribute to 'the simplicity and elegance of Garrod's interpretation of alcaptonuria and other inborn errors of metabolism as gene defects which resulted in inactivity of specific enzymes and thus in blocked reactions' (Beadle 1958).

CONSTITUTION, IDIOSYNCRASY, AND DIATHESIS

Man — and presumably lower animals had they been able to consider the problem — has known from earliest times that individuals have structural differences that may be inherited or acquired (a man may be born with only two fingers on one hand or may acquire this defect through disease or injury), and that they have chemical differences (many animals are attracted to the opposite sex by smell rather than by vision). Variation between individuals can be physical or chemical, genetic or acquired by contact with the environment. In medieval physiology, emphasis was placed on temperament, which was initially the relative proportions of the four cardinal humours (sanguine, choleric, phlegmatic, melancholic) which determined the individual's constitution. Constitution was then widened to be the individual's inborn qualities of body or mind that were inherited.

Constitution is therefore synonymous with genotype. An individual's genotype is altered by environmental factors, such as overeating or malnutrition, to determine the individual's phenotype. Early physicians, such as those of the Pythagorean school (who included Hippocrates (460–375 BC)), noticed that the effect of foods on individuals varied according to inborn susceptibility; it was also found that reactions to environmental factors could be acquired. Lucretius (c.95–55 BC) stated: 'Quod ali cibus est aliis fiat acre venenum' (What is food to one is fierce poison to others). This is idiosyncrasy, which we may define as an abnormal reaction to a stimulus, whether inborn or acquired, positive or negative; idiosyncrasies therefore include allergic reactions, and they can be acquired or lost. Garrod himself recorded (1931) that although he did not suffer from hay-fever, he was unable to stay in a room with the flowers of the orange-coloured buddleia without experiencing general discomfort and breathlessness; purple buddleia, however, had no such effect. A member of his family could not, when young, eat fish of the family Pleuronectidae (sole, plaice, turbot, halibut) without experiencing severe gastric symptoms; but from middle age onwards she lost this idiosyncrasy. Genotype and phenotype both affect susceptibility to disease; this susceptibility is diathesis, which we may define as a condition of the body, whether inborn or acquired, that causes it to be chronically predisposed to a certain disease. I have discussed on a previous occasion certain aspects of the history of these concepts (Sinclair 1962).

IMMUNOLOGY

Our knowledge of the mechanism of idiosyncrasies and diatheses has been greatly extended by recent advances in immunology, and we might be excused even a superficial excursion into this field had not connections with nutrition been very recently discovered. Mainly from work in Oxford by Gowans, we now know that immunity is produced through small lymphocytes which are of two types. T-lymphocytes, which are short-lived, are altered by the thymus, and are responsible for cell-mediated immunity. This is concerned with the rejection of transplants, with defence against neoplasms, with resistance to certain types of infection, and with some autoimmune processes. The thymus-altered lymphocytes respond to antigen by liberating non-antibody compounds generically termed 'lymphokines', and both enhance the phagocytic activity of macrophages and inhibit their migration. Ferber and Resch (1973) in Freiburg have shown that when lymphocytes are activated the palmitic acid in the 2-position of the phospholipids on their surface decreases and arachidonic acid greatly increases; free fatty acids appear on the surface and between lymphocytes, and may be the cytotoxic factor. Macrophages when activated release prostaglandins which inhibit activation of lymphocytes as does linoleic acid. B-lymphocytes, which are long-lived, arise in bone-marrow and are independent of the thymus. They are immunologically competent cells with immunological memory. They (or possibly large lymphocytes) give rise to plasmablasts which are converted into plasma cells which have a life-span of days and do not divide; these, activated by B-lymphocytes, produce immunoglobulins the chemistry of which has been elucidated by Porter, Professor of Biochemistry in Oxford. Immunoglobulins not only react with antigen; a small fraction of IgG, called cytophilic antibody, attaches itself to lipid receptors on the surfaces of macrophages which then become phagocytic (Fig. 1.1).

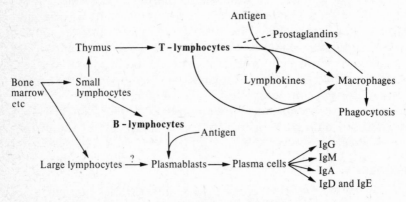

Fig. 1.1. Antigen, lymphocytes, and immunoglobulins.

We may mention three different aspects of immunology that concern nutrition. First, proteins or polypeptides from ingested foods may give rise to antibodies even in health. Sudden unexplained death in infancy, called 'cot death', may in some classes be caused by cow's milk antigens (Parish, Barrett, Coombs, Gunther, and Camps 1960). Work in Oxford 15 years ago demonstrated circulating antibodies to cow's milk protein and to gluten in the newborn (Wright, Taylor, Truelove, and Aschaffenburg 1962); cow's milk antibodies can also be shown in idiopathic steatorrhoea including coeliac disease (Taylor, Thomson, Truelove, and Wright 1961) and in ulcerative colitis (Taylor and Truelove 1961), and this disease can be provoked by milk (Truelove 1961). In coeliac disease and idiopathic steatorrhoea, there is an allergic response in the epithelial cells of the small-intestinal mucosa to a polypeptide of gliadin in wheat, as first indicated by Dicke and studied by Van der Kamer in the Netherlands.

A second interaction between immunity and nutrition concerns essential fatty acids (EFA), particularly the n-6 or linoleic (C18:2) class which includes arachidonic acid (C20:4). As mentioned above, when T-lymphocytes react with antigen their surface phospholipids lose palmitic acid (C16:0) in the 2-position and gain arachidonic acid; further, linoleic acid inhibits the activation of these lymphocytes by antigen. Also, EFA are the precursors of prostaglandins which are known to inhibit immune function; activated macrophages produce these and so cause a feedback inhibition of activation of lymphocytes. Another effect of EFA on immune function follows from their lowering in very-low-density-lipoprotein (VLDL) levels in plasma, since VLDL binds to lymphocytes and suppresses their immune reactions. Feeding milk supplemented with linoleic acid to babies vaccinated against measles raises antibody titres and shortens the duration of fever. The immunological or other role of EFA in multiple sclerosis is being very actively investigated at present, with various clinical trials in progress. Perhaps the most important part EFA play in immune responses, so far not investigated, might arise from the disorganized cellular membranes that occur in deficiency perhaps thereby assisting antigens to gain access to the surfaces of immune-responsive cells, and giving rise to autoimmune disease. The third interaction between immunity and nutrition is the effect of dietary deficiency on the production of T-lymphocytes and antibodies; since the latter are proteins it might be supposed that they would be deficient in kwashiorkor or protein-energy malnutirition (PEM), but this is not usually so. However, in PEM defects in cellular immunity may occur (Smythe *et al.* 1971).

This brief discussion has been mainly concerned with the individual's reaction to antigens. In the last five years the study of histocompatibility antigens (the HLA system) has greatly increased our knowledge of the susceptibility of individuals to environmental agents. The VIth human chromosome carries a cluster of genes that determine the structure of glycoproteins found on the surface of all nucleated cells of the body including platelets. These glycoproteins differ from one individual to another, and are the main antigenic barrier to transplantation of tissues between genetically non-identical individuals. They also regulate the immune response to a wide variety of antigens, mainly by affecting T-lymphocytes. Hence they affect the susceptibility to a variety of diseases. The HLA region of chromosome VI has about 1000 genes and four main loci: HLA-A,

−B, −C, and −D. The first three determine antigens that are present on the surfaces of all nucleated cells. Sometimes the association with susceptibility to disease is very strong: there is an association between HLA–B27 and ankylosing spondylitis in 95 per cent of patients. Enhanced resistance to disease may also be associated with the HLA system. Multiple sclerosis, which as mentioned above is connected with EFA, has been associated with various HLA factors, but recently has been found to be more strongly associated with an alloantigen on B–lymphocytes. Gluten-sensitive enteropathy is strongly associated with HLA–A1 and B8, and HLA–Bw35 appears to confer resistance.

FAVISM AND LATHYRISM

Lest it may appear that this brief discussion of the mode of inheritance of differences between individuals is irrelevant to nutrition, I mention two examples of diseases that can be produced by the broad bean, *Vicia faba*, whether raw or cooked. In the days of primitive medicine, half a century ago, Mühlens (1927) used one of the recently introduced derivatives of 8-aminoquinoline, namely plasmoquin, to treat the malaria he had intentionally induced in syphilitics as a pyrogen; he gave his patients a third disease, haemolytic anaemia, which in some was fatal. Eventually it was established that patients sensitive to 8-aminoquinolines, cases of favism, and some with non-spherocytic congenital haemolytic anaemia had deficiency in erythrocytes of glucose 6-phosphate dehydrogenase (G6PD). Of this condition there are various types: the A⁻ and A+ types found mainly in negroes, the Mediterranean type, the Canton type in some south Chinese, and others admirably standardized by the WHO ten years ago. Most patients with the Mediterranean type have no clinical signs or symptoms unless they encounter certain drugs or broad beans or infections; but some develop haemolytic crises without known inciting cause, and haemolytic disease of the newborn may occur. Favism is not merely deficiency of G6PD in erythrocytes, since most negroes with the A⁻ type have this deficiency but can eat broad beans with impunity, and in some cases it has been shown that [51] Cr-labelled deficient erythrocytes are not destroyed when the beans are eaten; apparently favism requires an additional genetic defect. The enzyme converts glucose 6-phosphate to 6-phosphogluconate, generating NADPH from NADP; NADPH produces GSH from oxidized glutathione, and the former is essential for erythrocyte survival. The disease is inherited as a sex-linked trait; and it appears to confer some protection against falciparum malaria, probably because the parasite requires GSH for optimal growth. In broad beans the principle responsible for favism appears to be the nucleoside vicine, which is the only natural nucleoside known to contain a glucose residue.

Broad beans can also produce lathyrism, which is a very different disease. It occurs mainly in India and the Mediterranean area where peas of the genus *Lathyrus* are eaten. There are two forms of the disease according as the nervous system or skeleton is affected. It appears that the aminoacid asparagine can be dehydrated to β-cyanoalanine which is then reduced to α, γ-diaminobutyric acid, and both of these are neurolathyrogens in lower animals as is α, β-diaminopropionic acid which could arise from asparagine by a Hoffman degradation. On the other hand, β-cyanoalanine can be decarboxylated to give β-aminopropionitrile which appears to be the osteolathyrogen.

THE NORMAL INDIVIDUAL

Usually we consider the 'normal' individual of a given category of sex, age, activity, and environment. But what is the normal individual? I considered this problem in a review of the assessment of human nutriture (Sinclair 1948) and may here summarize the three distinct concepts. The first is that of perfection: a normal individual is one who is perfect according to some arbitrary set of standards. But we cannot accept this definition because what is optimum in one set of circumstances may be disadvantageous in another: deficiency of thiamine increases the resistance of the body to an attack of poliomyelitis. The second is the concept of pathology according to which an individual is normal who is free from the signs and symptoms of active disease but may have mild imperfections of the body. The physician's examination is too crude to establish normality: severe depletion of body calcium may be present for a long period before signs or symptoms of osteomalacia appear; deficiency of G6PD in erythrocytes may be undetected until the individual eats broad beans or is given an antimalarial drug; another inborn error of metabolism (one of the four originally described by Garrod) is congenital pentosuria in which there is a defect in the conversion of L-xylulose to xylitol, and this appears to be harmless. Thirdly, the statistical concept of normality has to draw an arbitrary line between normal and abnormal. If a variate in a homogeneous population follows a Gaussian distribution curve, about 95 per cent of the individuals will fall within plus or minus twice the standard deviation. In a Caucasian population (but not a Mongoloid on traditional diets) dental caries, atheroma, and (in adolescence) acne vulgaris would probably be considered normal.

It is necessary to adopt a statistical definition of normality on occasion, for instance in specifying heights of individuals in a stated population. But unless thus specified normality is best defined in physiological terms: the condition of the body, or of some part or function of the body, is normal when it allows the usual functions to be adequately performed in the usual environment. Normal body-weight is not so straightforward as height. There has been a tendency to regard the readily achieved maximum weight of children as the optimum, and when US children enter a swimming-pool tidal waves are produced. We know from the work of Clive McCay and others (1939) on a variety of lower animals that overnutrition during the period before maturity (which can be regarded as the onset of ability to reproduce) hastens maturity and causes earlier death from chronic degenerative diseases. My colleague Dr Dagmar Wilson showed that maturity occurred earlier in Oxford girls than in Nigerian, and in Britain over the years the age at which maturity is reached has greatly decreased. We customarily attribute this to 'better' nutrition, but it may partly be harmful overnutrition. Undernutrition and malnutrition cause paradoxes in body-weight. The infant suffering from kwashiorkor may be overweight because deficiency of protein causes low colloid osmotic pressure of plasma and so an increase in extracellular fluid. Undernutrition in adults is usually accompanied by increase in extracellular fluid probably through adrenal cortical activity, and gross oedema may occur. More commonly, body-weight may be very deceptive since bone and muscle weigh more than an equal volume of fat; the mesomorphic athlete in training with little adipose tissue may weigh much more than an obese endomorph of the same height.

MAN-VALUES AND WOMAN-VALUES

Global nutrition is the most important problem facing mankind as populations increase, food decreases and there are serious nutritional problems in all countries whether developed or emerging. In considering this problem we need to scan a very much wider field than that provided by the differences between individuals. In our broad sweep we must consider the average individual. Who is he or she?

When, largely as a result of Liebig (1803–73), analyses of foods became available a century ago, human requirements were initially guessed in terms of what a person in health was actually eating. This might be a reasonable approximation for energy, but with protein and especially calcium absurd conclusions could be drawn. Refinements of chemistry and advances in physiology permitted balances to be done. After the turn of the century excellent requirements of energy were formulated, of which the classical ones in this country were produced during the First World War when at the end of 1916 the British had lost more than 2 million tons of shipping through German submarines, and an incompetent Trade Minister announced (17 October 1916) that 'We want to avoid any rationing of our people in food' and resigned to be replaced by a disastrous Minister of Food. The Royal Society had set up in 1915 a Food (War) Committee which included scientists of the distinction of Gowland Hopkins. Reporting in December 1916, it concluded:

A full consideration of the dietary requirements of a nation for the most part engaged in active work has convinced the Committee that these requirements cannot be satisfactorily met on a less supply in the food as purchased than 100 grammes protein, 100 grammes fat, 500 grammes carbohydrate, equal approximately to 3,400 calories per 'man' per day, a 'man' being an average workman doing an average day's work (Royal Society 1916).

It matters little that they misused Rubner's factors, and we can criticize the actual figures. The important point is that here scientific knowledge was being accurately applied to the solution of an important problem in public health that was being mismanaged by ignorant politicians.

These figures were, as stated, for the average man engaged in moderate work. He was the individual first selected as a standard at the beginning of the century by Atwater, who probably did better work with clearer insight upon energy than anyone before or since (Atwater and Bryant 1900). Atwater coefficients for energy requirements allowed his moderately active man 3500 kcal (14.65 MJ). This was not the first system of coefficients; Engel in 1895 had produced a 'Quet' scale (named in memory of the Belgian statistician Quételet) for consumption in general within the family, the unit being the newborn child; the adult man and woman were allowed 3.5 and 3.0 respectively. In 1932 a Commission of the Health Organization of the League of Nations produced a new set of coefficients, now allowing their unit, the average man, 2700 net kcal (11.3 MJ) or 3000 gross (12.6 MJ). The last proposal of this organization, upon which so many people bestowed so much hope, was produced by its Technical Commission in 1938; the two distinguished secretaries have recently died, Dame Harriette Chick, at the age of 102, and Professor Bigwood. The Commission's allowances for energy (taking into account sex, age, and activity) were admirably conceived, although trivial criticisms could be made: a male or female who had reached the nineteenth but not the twentieth birthday was omitted, and pregnant women received the same allowance as non-pregnant.

During the Second World War the Oxford Nutrition Survey drew up its own allowances for energy and nutrients, which were published (Malnutrition, 1948) and largely adopted (except for protein) by the

Committee on Nutrition of the British Medical Association in 1950. We used the moderately active woman as the unit because her requirements were in general the mean of those of the population. And we introduced a nutritional unit, the Atwater, which enormously simplified food tables (Sinclair 1949). This gave a visual check to the accuracy of dietary computations, and obviated the mental gymnastics of jumping between thousands of calories or units of vitamin A, hundreds of grams of carbohydrate or units of vitamin D, tens of grams of protein, tens of milligrams of ascorbic acid, milligrams of thiamine, micrograms of vitamin B_{12}.

From 1943 onwards the Food and Nutrition Board of the National Research Council in Washington, D.C., has published *Recommended dietary allowances*. It is specifically stated that 'The recommendations are not requirements, since they represent, not merely minimal needs of average persons, but nutrient levels selected to cover individual variations in a substantial majority of the population.' Yet it is stated 'that caloric allowances must be adjusted up or down to meet specific needs' which can hardly be correct if 'the allowance levels are considered to cover individual variations among normal persons as they live in the United States subjected to ordinary environmental stresses'. The Report of the Committee of the British Medical Association aimed, as had the Oxford Nutrition Survey, to provide values that applied to the average individual in a specified category. At the same time the Canadian Council on Nutrition (1950) produced very different standards which represented 'a nutritional floor beneath which maintenance of the health of the people cannot be assumed'. The FAO Committee on Calorie Requirements (1950) 'has throughout considered requirements *at the physiological level*. The figures put forward relate to the food as consumed.' This is a contradiction: as Atwater so clearly showed, the energy in food as eaten is not that which is physiologically available, because of losses in digestion (both unabsorbed energy and energy in Atwater's 'metabolic products') and in the urine. This error was repeated word for word in the Second Report (FAO 1957). Since it is almost impossible to assess what foods people do eat and to translate such crude assessments into aliments and nutrients, the accuracy of yardsticks of requirements or allowances is perhaps not essential.

The coefficients used for comparing the requirements or allowances of individuals of different sex or age or activity, whether we take as unity the moderately active man or woman or the newborn infant, will alter according to which nutritional factor we are considering. Adolescent boys need more energy and protein than do

adult men of the same physical activity; during the period of repro-
ductive activity men may need about seven times as much EFA as
corresponding women (judged by work on lower animals), but less
iron; during lactation women need disproportionately large amounts
of calcium. It is usual in family dietary studies to assume that the
food available is allocated according to the individual needs of
energy; but we found in the famine in the western Netherlands in
1945 that although the adult male in a family would travel long
distances to scavenge for food, this when obtained was divided
equally between all members of the family including young children.
Compassion overcame reason.

SOME FACTORS AFFECTING AN INDIVIDUAL'S NUTRITIONAL
REQUIREMENTS

It is probable that water is the only single chemical compound
essential in the diet; the body does not make sufficient to replenish
losses. Ascorbic acid can be replaced by an analogue such as the
gluco-ascorbic acid; the essential amino-acids can probably be replaced by the corresponding keto-acids. But not all forms of a
nutrient have equal activity. Further, for reasons usually unknown,
some individuals have greatly increased requirements while others
are unusually susceptible to toxicity from excess. Some of these
problems of nutritional individuality were discussed by Roger
Williams (1956). Twenty-three years ago it was found that some
infants developed convulsions because they had very large requirements of pyridoxine; therefore they fail to make sufficient of the
inhibitory compound γ-aminobutyric acid which is formed in the
brain by glutamate decarboxylase of which pyridoxal phosphate
is coenzyme. Then certain patients with microcytic hypochromic
anaemia were found to respond to large amounts of pyridoxine,
about seven times the usual requirement; it appeared there was some
inherited abnormality in the metabolism of the vitamin which is
needed as a coenzyme in the condensation of glycine and succinyl-
CoA to form δ-aminolevulinic acid in the synthesis of haeme. It is
stated that women taking the contraceptive pill may have their
requirements of pyridoxine increased at least tenfold, which led
György (1971) to increase the supposed daily requirement by a
factor of more than ten to 25 mg. Occasional individuals require
large amounts of nicotinic acid despite high intake of trytophan:
I encountered a farmer's wife whose apparently adequate diet
included considerable quantities of milk, yet she was certified insane
and only when she sat in the sun and developed a skin rash that did
not respond to the usual ointments was the possibility of pellagra

considered; her psychosis cleared with oral nicotinic acid. On the other hand, infantile hypercalcaemia is caused by unusual susceptibility to the toxicity of vitamin D; I found that deficiency of EFA causes this increased susceptibility, and I believe feeding dried cow's milk fortified with normally non-toxic amounts of the vitamin caused the disease. Recently the genetic abnormality in infants that causes vitamin-D-resistant rickets has been elucidated through work of DeLuca, Kodicek, and others. Ultraviolet light converts in the skin 7-dehydrocholesterol to cholecalciferol which in the liver is hydroxylated in the 25-position and then further hydroxylated in the kidney to give 1,25-dihydroxycholecalciferol. The final step is decreased in these infants, and of course it is missing in patients who have lost renal function and are kept alive by dialysis.

Adaptation to different dietary conditions is a subject that is becoming clearer. Chronic alcoholics can oxidize much larger amounts of alcohol in a given time than those not used to it; alcohol increases the smooth endoplasmic reticulum of the hepatic microsomes and so increases the cytochrome P_{450} system; this system is induced by drugs such as phenobarbital, and is very important in hydroxylating these and carcinogens such as methylcholanthrene and 3,4-benzpyrene. Since therefore alcohol increases the ability of the body to deal with certain toxins, some might regard it as a nutrient. A man who for sixty years drank a quart of Scotch whisky daily managed a successful business almost until his death at the age of 93. The familiar adaptation to dietary deficiency of calcium is obscure, but A.R.P. Walker (Walker, Fox, and Irving 1948) demonstrated adaptation to dietary phytase, the enzyme in whole-grain cereals that is believed to be responsible for the deficiency of zinc in poor Sudanese boys, though why they respond with stunted growth more than girls is not explained. Vegans may adapt to their diet deficient in vitamin B_{12} by increased synthesis of the vitamin by the intestinal flora, as in other strict herbivores; but this may be more a case of natural selection since if they do not obtain the vitamin in this way and do not take a supplement they die.

Eskimos are particularly interesting in view of their carnivorous diet very low in linoleic acid and other members of the n-6 family, low in linolenic acid but relatively very high in C20:5 and C22:6 of this family (n-3). They do not get the skin lesions that might be expected, and they have no thrombotic episodes such as ischaemic heart disease despite presumably having very low prostacyclin (PGI_2) which Vane and his colleagues (Moncada, Gryglewski, Bunting, and Vane 1976) discovered is the most active known antithrombotic agent; but the thromboxanes formed from C20:5n-3 do not aggregate platelets (Needleman, Minkes, and Raz 1976). Very recently Vane and his colleagues with my Danish colleagues have found that C20:5n-3 also gives rise to prostacyclin (PGI$_3$) which is extremely active in disaggregating platelets (Dyerberg, Bang, Stoffersen, Moncada, and Vane 1978). Figure 1.2 summarizes recent work in this interesting field.

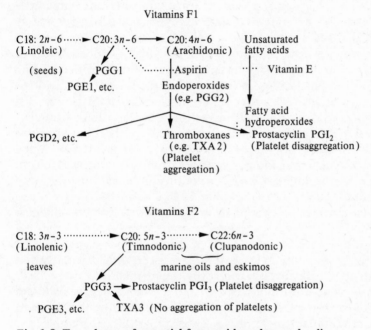

Fig. 1.2. Two classes of essential fatty acids and prostglandins.

We do not know why eskimos do not get scurvy despite a diet low in ascorbic acid, the only good source of which appears to be seal liver. They do not get ketosis despite very high dietary fat, and this is not adaptation; polyunsaturated fatty acids do not produce ketosis, and I suggested this might arise from γ-oxidation. An interesting problem of possible adaptation in Eskimos concerns docosamonoenoic fatty acids. It is well established that erucic acid (C22:1n-9) produces myocardial fibrosis in animals, and in Canada a strain of rape seed almost free of this fatty acid has been developed. More recently its isomer, cetoleic acid (C22:1n-11), has been found to be as or more toxic, and this is the main fatty acid in various fish (12 per cent in herring; 9 per cent in salmon). Eskimos and seals have large amounts of this fatty acid in their diets and therefore their bodies (6 per cent in seal oil), but seals do not show the heart lesions nor apparently do Eskimos. Since both obtain large amounts during foetal life and from birth in milk, it is possible that their cardiac muscle mitochondria adapt to it and oxidize it. Further, carnivores such as cats obtain arachidonic acid in their diets and have lost the ability to form it from linoleic acid (Rivers *et al.* 1976); Eskimos may have a similar disability.

There are problems concerning vitamin A in different individuals which are still not understood. I have experienced, as had previously Hecht and also Wald, that sometimes volunteers starting on a diet free of the vitamin and carotenoids will go for the expected year or so before any diminution occurs in the final rod threshold of the dark-adapted eye ('night-blindness'); at other times similar individuals on the same diet show significant diminution in about five weeks, as I have discussed elsewhere (Rodgers and Sinclair 1969). Deficient infants develop xerophthalmia often after their mothers have noticed night-blindness, and this was well studied by Bloch (1921) in the First World War when economic considerations caused the Danes to export their butter, and margarine was not supplemented; but in the famine in the western Netherlands in 1945 I saw a number of such infants whom Professor Jonxis had in his wards in Rotterdam, some of whom died of pneumonia following atelectasis caused by desquamation of the bronchial epithelium. We do not know why—if it be correct—vitamin A protects against lung cancer. A particularly important aspect of vitamin A, which we do understand, is that taboos sometimes prevent individuals eating rich sources, such as fish, and endemic blindness occurs, as in parts of Africa; this is an urgent problem in nutritional education.

Individual requirements of nutrients are also affected by the interrelations between them. Obviously requirements of thiamine are related to dietary carbohydrate since as Peters first showed in Oxford (cf. Peters 1936) the vitamin is needed for oxidation of pyruvate; similarly with pyridoxine and dietary protein, and presumably pantothenic acid and dietary fat. There are relations between trace elements, for instance copper with zinc and with molybdenum. A very important interrelationship recently discovered by workers in the National Nutrition Institute in Hyderabad concerns pellagra. Belavardy and her colleagues (1963) have established that leucine (which is high in sorghum and ordinary maize but low in opaque 2) inhibits the synthesis of NAD from nicotinic acid and so promotes pellagra whereas isoleucine interferes with the absorption of leucine in the gut; therefore dietary factors promoting pellagra are low nicotinic acid, low tryptophan, low isoleucine, and high leucine.

Deficiency of tryptophan in the body can occur for another reason: in Hartnup disease it, as well as certain other amino-acids, is lost in the urine and inadequately absorbed in the intestine, and therefore signs of pellagra appear. This is a rare inborn error of metabolism.

A very common alteration in the intestine concerns lactase. Congenital lactase deficiency is fortunately rare since almost all milks contain lactose. But in most mammals lactase disappears after late infancy, milk not being a natural adult food. This occurs in Asians and most Africans, although not in most Caucasians and in those African tribes that traditionally drink milk. Therefore intolerance to milk is very common in adult life.

Finally, there are differences in requirements of nutrients for protection against acute deficiency and production of full health. We know that 6.5 mg daily of ascorbic acid will cure clinical scurvy (Hodges *et al.* 1971); but it is possible, though as yet unproved, that much larger amounts are needed for full protection against certain infections. We know from infants and adults given intravenous fat-free alimentation that about 4 per cent of the energy as linoleic acid will prevent acute EFA-deficiency; but for maximum protection of platelets against aggregation Vergroesen (1973) has suggested that between 12 and 16 per cent is needed. Acute and chronic deficiencies are very different. An acute deficiency is produced suddenly and usually results either in cure after therapy or death. A chronic deficiency lasts for a long time and therefore of necessity is mild. Acute deficiency of EFA undoubtedly causes skin lesions in adults and infants, and in the latter failure of growth and increased susceptibility to infections; I believe that a chronic relative deficiency (which means a low ratio in the body of EFA to non-EFA such as long-chain saturated fatty acids) causes faulty structure of cellular membranes (such as plasma, mitochondrial, lysosomal) so that the cells of the body are more susceptible to a variety of insults; and mainly for this reason various chronic degenerative diseases are increasingly prevalent in developed countries and are starting to appear in Japan and in the emerging countries in which there are such widespread nutritional problems of an entirely different kind.

CONCLUSION

At the World Food Council in Rome in June 1975 Dr Boerma, the Director-General of the FAO, declared that the FAO's aim of eradicating world hunger in ten years cannot be achieved, and the situation will become worse; a French agricultural economist stated that the biggest famine in world history had just begun. The 'green revolution' has faltered since the wrong crops have been grown, the wrong soil cultivated, and policy dictated by ignorant officials. We need urgently to produce more food and to improve our knowledge of the food we do produce. This food must be planned to supply nationally and internationally the nutritional needs of man which must be based on the average individual. The genes produce the soil for the production of the individual whose constitution, diathesis, and idiosyncracies arise partly from these and partly from environmental factors such as nutrition. The physician is concerned with the individual, but public health is concerned with families constituting societies, as Dr Ghassemi discusses in a following paper. The societies are ultimately grouped into nations which together constitute the world community. For this our forlorn aim is Freedom from Want, which in our context means freedom from want of those foods acceptable to peoples with different traditions and supplying the aliments and nutrients needed by each individual according to variable requirements.

Tradition is important. Our theme is nutritional education. The public must be advised within the context of what is acceptable and what is practical. Food habits can be changed, sometimes for the worse as has now happened amongst almost all Eskimos, sometimes for the better as was shown before the Second World War by the 'Oslo breakfast', and very recently by the decline in ischaemic heart disease in north Belgium as compared with the south, apparently through better education in the former to substitute butter with margarine (Joossens *et al.* 1977). Education should be based upon established scientific facts, but these are disappointingly few because so little support is given to human nutritional research. When facts are not available common sense must be used since we cannot wait for scientific proof before advising upon the urgent nutritional problems that confront us. The family doctor should be a source of advice, but almost no nutrition is taught to medical students as I emphasized in my paper on this subject for the First World Conference on Medical Education in 1954; my plea was unproductive. Dietists, social workers, and the radio and television are all important; but these are luxuries not available to the masses of the world amongst whom the most urgent problems exist. So this Congress on Nutritional Education had much to attempt.

REFERENCES

Atwater, W.O. and Bryant, A.P. (1900). The availability and fuel value of food material. *Rep. Storrs agric.Exp.Sta.* 1899, p. 73.

Beadle, G.W. (1958). Genes and chemical reactions in *Neurospora. Nobel lectures, physiology or medicine*, p. 587. Elsevier, Amsterdam.

Belavardy, B., Srikantia, S.G., and Pearson, W.N. (1963). Leucine and pellagra, *Lancet*, i, 778.

Bloch, C.E. (1921). Clinical investigation of xerophthalmia and dystrophy in infants and young children. *J.Hyg.,Camb.* **19**, 283.
British Medical Association (1950). *Report of the Committee on Nutrition.* BMA, London.
Canadian Council on Nutrition (1950). *A dietary standard for Canada. Nutr.* **2**, 6.
Dyerberg, J., Bang, H.O., Stoffersen, E., Moncada, S., and Vane, J.R. (1978). Eicosapentaenoic acid and prevention of thrombosis and atherosclerosis?'. *Lancet* ii, 117.
Engel, E. (1895). *Die Lebenskosten belgischer Arbeiter-Familien früher und ietzt. Bull.int.Inst.Stat.* **9**, 1.
Ferber, E. and Resch, K. (1973). Phospholipid metabolism of stimulated lymphocytes: activation of acyl-CoA:lysolecithin acyl-transferases in microsomal membranes. *Biochim.Biophys.Acta* **296**, 335.
Food and Agriculture Organization (1950). *Calorie requirements.* FAO Washington, D.C.
— (1957). *Calorie requirements.* FAO, Rome.
Garrod, A.E. (1902). The incidence of alcaptonuria: a study in chemical individuality. *Lancet* ii, 1616.
— (1909). *Inborn errors of metabolism.* Frowde, Hodder and Stoughton, London.
— (1931). *The inborn factors in disease. An essay.* Clarendon Press, Oxford.
— (1923). *Inborn errors of metabolism* (2nd edn). Frowde, Hodder & Stoughton, London.
György, P. (1971). Developments leading to the metabolic role of vitamin B_6. *Am.J.clin.Nutr.* **24**, 1250.
Hodges, R.E., Hood, J., Canham, J.E., Sauberlich, H.E., and Baker, E.M. (1971). Clinical manifestations of ascorbic acid deficiency in man. *Am.J.clin.Nutr.* **24**, 432.
Joossens, J.V. *et al.* (1977). The pattern of food and mortality in Belgium. *Lancet* i, 1069.
Landsteiner, K. (1900). Zur Kenntniss der antifermativen, lytischen und agglutinierenden Wirkungen des Blutserums und der Lymphe. *Zbl.Bakt.* **27**, 357.
League of Nations, Conference of Experts (1932). Standardisation of certain methods used in making dietary studies. *Bull.Hlth Org.* **1**, 477.
League of Nations, Technical Commission on Nutrition (1938). Report on the work of its third session. *Bull.Hlth Org.* **7**, 461.
McCay, C.M., Maynard, L.A., Sperling, G., and Barnes, L.L. (1939). Retarded growth, life span, ultimate body size and age changes in the albino rat after feeding diets restricted in calories. *J.Nutr.* **18**, 1.
Malnutrition and Starvation in the Western Netherlands (1948). The Hague: General State Printing Office, Part II, p. 269.
Moncada, S., Gryglewski, R.J., Bunting, S., and Vane, J.R. (1976). An enzyme isolated from arteries transforms prostaglandin endoperoxides to an unstable substance that inhibits platelet aggregation. *Nature* **262**, 663.
Mühlens, P. (1927). Die Behandlung der naturlichen menschlichen Malaria-infektion mit Plasmochin. *Naturwiss.* **15**, 1162.
National Research Council, Food and Nutrition Board (1943). *Recommended dietary allowances.* National Research Council, Washington, D.C.
Needleman, P., Minkes, M., and Raz, A. (1976). Thromboxanes: selective biosynthesis and distinct biological properties. *Science* **193**, 163.
Parish, W.E., Barrett, A.M., Coombs, R.R., Gunther, M., and Camps, (1960). Hypersensitivity to milk and sudden death in infancy. *Lancet* ii, 1106.

Peters, R.A. (1936). The biochemical lesions in vitamin B_1 deficiency. *Lancet* i, 1161.

Rivers, J.P.W., Sinclair, A.J., and Crawford, M.A. (1975). Inability of the cat to desaturate essential fatty acids. *Nature* 258, 171.

Rodgers, F.C. and Sinclair, H.M. (1969). *Metabolic and nutritional eye diseases.* Thomas, Springfield, Ill.

Royal Society (1916). *The food supply of the United Kingdom. A report drawn up by a committee of the Royal Society at the request of the President of the Board of Trade.* Cd 12219. HMSO, London.

Sinclair, H.M. (1948). The assessment of human nutriture. *Vitamin Horm.* 6, 102.

—— (1949). The Atwater—a nutritional unit. *Brit. J. Nutr.* 3, x.

—— (1954). The teaching of nutrition. *Proc. 1st World Conf. Med. Educ.* p. 717. Oxford University Press, London.

—— (1962). Historical aspects of inborn errors of metabolism. *Proc. Nutr. Soc.* 21, 1.

Smythe, P.M., Schonland, M., Brereton-Stiles, G.C., Coovadia, H.M., Grace, H.J., Loening, W.E.K., Mafoyane, A., Parent, M.A., and Vos, G.H. (1971). Thymolymphatic deficiency and depression of cell-mediated immunity in protein-calorie malnutrition. *Lancet* ii, 939.

Taylor, K.B., Thomson, D.L., Truelove, S.C., and Wright, R. (1961). An immunological study of coeliac disease and idiopathic steatorrhoea. *Br. med. J.* ii, 1727.

—— and Truelove, S.C. (1961). Circulation antibodies to milk proteins in ulcerative colitis. *Br. med. J.* ii, 924.

Truelove, S.C. (1961). Ulcerative colitis provoked by milk. *Br. med. J.* i, 154.

Vergroesen, A.J. (1973). Therapeutic effects of linoleic acid. In *4th Nutricia Sympos., Groningen 9-11 May*, pp. 55-64 (ed. Jonxis, Visser, and Troelstra). Stenfert Kroeve B.V., Leiden.

Walker, A.R.P., Fox, F.W., and Irving, J.T. (1948). Studies in human mineral metabolism: the effect of bread rich in phytate phosphorus on metabolism of certain mineral salts with special reference to calcium. *Biochem J.* 42, 452.

Williams, R.J. (1956). *Biochemical individuality.* Chapman & Hall, London.

Wilson, D.C. and Sutherland, I. (1953). The age of the menarche in the tropics. *Br. med. J.* ii, 607.

Wright, R., Taylor, K.B., Truelove, S.C., and Aschaffenburg, R. (1962). Circulating antibodies to cow's milk proteins and gluten in the newborn. *Br. med. J.* ii, 513.

2 Nutrition in relation to
the family and the community
M. CÉPÈDE

Galen (AD 131–201) when claiming to be able to modify his patients' behaviour by prescribing certain diets obviously dealt with individuals. Brillat-Savarin (1755–1826) when writing: 'Tell me what you eat and I will tell you what you are', went further and may have been considering the way of life of different ethnic groups. A few years later, von Feuerbach (1804–1872) playing with words and stressing: 'Man ist, was er isst' (Man is what he eats), evidently had ethno-sociological preoccupations.

Cultural aspects of eating were stressed in the lecture delivered by Jean Trémolières to the International Congress of Nutrition (Trémolières 1969). He was advising against any foreign model of food change imposed on people and went as far as to assert that man chooses the food which will make him the kind of man he wants to be! Such affirmation appears to be too optimistic. Food habits in no way belong to a field of freedom for man. They are determined by traditions which, too often, have been imposed by present or historic domination (Cépède 1970). Food is a social phenomenon.

A few preliminary remarks are necessary about the measurement of food consumption by groups. Multiplying the nutritionist's prescription by the number in the population will only lead to undernutrition. Professor Hugh Sinclair (Ch. 1) draws our attention to the differences between the United States, Canadian, and British 'norms'. A controversy has arisen recently between the WHO/FAO Expert Committee and the Protein Advisory Groups of the United Nations on caloric and protein requirements. Each group spoke a different language! The Expert Committee aimed at measuring the needs of a population in good health, living in an adequate environment while the Protein Advisory Group (PAG) aimed at determining what a population should eat when it is living in an unfavourable environment (with endemic parasitic infestations and sickness) to maintain and, if possible, to improve its health conditions. When protein (and iron) requirements are in question there is little wonder that PAG recommendations are far above those of the Expert Committee.

Public opinion is surprised by such controversaries and is in danger of losing faith in science, or at least in scientists. Nevertheless any property under consideration must always be clarified by careful definition. Measurements are, indeed, necessary but measurements can be misleading. One cannot deal with a population without taking into consideration its composition, for example its age-classes, vulnerable groups, and manual workers—each group with its own particular needs.

If only the caloric requirements are under consideration it may be concluded that a population with a high proportion of young people needs less food than an older one. But if one takes into account the food of animal origin required in the diet for the growth and development of man's offspring the conclusion is quite different. Lengelle and Cépède (1953) calculated that the requirements per caput in Egypt were 1 per cent greater than those in France. On repeating the calculations again in 1962 (Cépède 1962) on three population models we obtained figures of 6028 'vegetable' calories for the economically developed population and 6009 and 6029 respectively for the two developing population models, the first being assumed to be stable and the second to be in demographic expansion.

It is also necessary to remember that simply to satisfy average requirements per caput is usually insufficient. For example, an inquiry in the mountain villages of the Swiss Alps revealed that when the food supply was equal to 100 per cent of the average requirements, 60 per cent of the population received in fact less than 90 per cent of its own needs. Such inequalities might be even greater in other regions.

Sociologists as well as politicians must take into account inequalities in actual consumption, in particular prestige consumption and waste production. Points such as these led a group of French nutritionists (Richet and Mans 1965) to conclude, 'In order to have enough, one has to have too much.'

From the above calculations it seems that a food diet of about 6000 'vegetable' calories per caput per day, that is 2400 calories of which 500 are of animal origin, can satisfy both caloric and specific needs (Castro 1952).

When food consumption level is low—or has been low for a long period—those who can afford to do so often eat much more than is necessary. A dimorphism between an obese ruling class and an undernourished populace appears to me to be one of the most obvious signs of a hungry country. If we look at nineteenth- and early twentieth-century family portraits in the developed countries when only the well-to-do could afford such memorials of themselves, the signs of *embonpoint* are plain to see. Only when an awareness of having conquered hunger spreads throughout the best-fed countries of the world does class dimorphism disappear and the unemployed worker becomes indistinguishable from the millionaire when they lie side by side on the beach.

Keeping such remarks in mind we turn now to some aspects of food as a social phenomenon. Man, recognized to be an omnivorous animal, appears as carnivorous by tendency and vegetarian under constraints.

In the market-oriented society in which we are living food inequalities under economic constraints are obvious between rich and poor. It goes so far that the majority of the 'undernourished' are found today in the families of food producers. In Macedonia, in the middle of the so-called 'over-production' depression, the small children of the dairy producers suffered severely from malnutrition due to lack of milk. The reason was that the price paid for milk was so low that the last drop had to be sold on the market to obtain the necessary monetary resources indispensable for the family's survival. The old Benin man's saying, 'Thank God for not having given to man the power to allocate air to those whom he likes', was perfectly right. Otherwise no one would have survived.

Economic constraints may be considered as causes of some of the diseases which affect those who are only a little better off than the poorest. Beriberi and pellagra are two examples of such diseases. Those who have stopped consuming brown rice ('wild man's rice') before they can afford to buy the supplementary foods that make Indonesian and Chinese meals so nutritious are in danger of beriberi. Similarly those who, formerly in Europe and now in Africa, have shifted from millet to maize have demonstrated the danger of developing pellagra if they are not able to pay for complementary vitamins and proteins.

When analysing the findings of the first World Food Survey in 1934–8 one of the most obvious statistical 'laws' was that the consumption of pulses, not only as a percentage but also as an absolute quantity, tends to fall as food consumption rises. Also the previously accepted idea that the total protein in the diet was constant is actually belied by the facts found in urban populations in African towns. Families recently arrived from their villages are ceasing to eat pulses and millet long before they have the purchasing power to obtain even a small amount of meat. The percentage of protein in the diet is, in fact, below what we have been led to believe is essential.

On the other hand, since the emergence of the 'law' noted in the 1934–8 survey, it has become obvious that the most affluent classes of the rich countries are increasing their consumption of pulses to a surprising extent. Such facts run counter to what is expected on general grounds.

Eating traditions may derive also from non-economic constraints. Among the poor of both the Third World and the industrialized countries the status attaching to the consumption of meat means that it is kept for the head of the family (usually the person who could best do without it) while those needing it most—children, adolescents, pregnant women, and nursing mothers—go short.

Meat is only one example. In 1271 Marco Polo wrote, 'Among the Tartars only the Great Khan's family and, by a special decision of Gengis Khan, the Ouirates were allowed to use mare's milk' (Dido 1865). Such traditions had nothing to do with economic considerations. Food habits are cultural traits in every society.

Hunters eat game meat, fishermen eat fish, cattle raisers eat dairy products and sometimes meat, peasants eat vegetable foods, and such facts are only obvious consequences of their way of life in their own environment. Their morphological as well as cultural differences are evidently affected by such food habits. For example in Kenya the dimorphism between Kikuyus and Masai is a classical instance. But the resources available from the milieu do not give a complete explanation of food habits. The fish consumption by some populations living near the coast of South America is low even when fish are plentiful but, by contrast, stockfish (dried cod) is a traditional dish in the mountains of Central France.

The recent explosive development of fisheries in the south-east Pacific Ocean—in which the FAO has taken a large part—did not change the situation there, because anchovies from Peru, the premier country in fisheries in the region, are processed into fish meal for export as cattle food while protein hunger is severe for local people.

Religious traditions also exert an influence on food habits. The Christian obligation to abstain regularly from eating meat is responsible for the tradition of importing dried cod into Central France. Iberic peoples have for centuries been dominated by Moslems. In order to force Christians to identify themselves the rulers offered them meat on days of abstinence. Spaniards and Portuguese are strict observers and many would have preferred death to sin. But the Church, as is well known, 'does not wish for the death of a sinner', and even less the death of the faithful. So by a Papal Bull the Iberic people were granted the privilege of not complying with the prescribed abstinence. Latin America, having been colonized and Christianized by the Spanish and Portuguese conquistadores, had the privilege extended to them also.

In considering resistance to change in food habits, fact-finding is not enough. It is necessary to understand the motivations. People are conscious of the fact that food habits result from long experience.

The original motivations behind the rules may have been forgotten but, obscure as it may be, a memory makes people feel strongly that the rules had been wisely established and to transgress them would be dangerous.

'Aliens' food is not good for us', they affirm, and it may be true. The actual intestinal flora of a population results from its traditional food habits and it might react unfavourably to a change in diet. Professor Raw (Ch. 10) recalls the problems arising with certain populations which have a lactase deficiency. Undoubtedly every human infant has enough lactase to enable him to utilize his mother's milk. If Caucasian students in America as well as African cattle-rearing groups have retained, as adults, their ability to produce lactase while other ethnic groups lose this ability the matter need not be unduly surprising. To describe as 'normal' the American adult of Caucasian origin or to see him as *nourrison prolongé*, is another matter.

Even if proposed new foods are harmless people know that food is a factor in their identity. Sometimes they will maintain this view-point stressing, 'We do not want to become *them*, we want to remain ourselves.'

Special consideration needs to be given to such negative habits as 'prohibited' or 'taboo' foods, which are often quoted by irritated nutrition educators. Such prohibitions are more frequent against eating foods of animal origin than of vegetable origin. This can be because eating animal products implies crime—a living animal has to be killed for its flesh. Eating eggs is also destruction of life. Drinking milk means that a young animal has to be deprived of its mother's milk. Blood is often labelled 'impure' and slaughtering ritual by Hebrews and Moslems for example is designed to eliminate blood from meat. Cooking, particularly hot cooking, may have been a desacralization ritual.

Health considerations are often quoted in order to justify prohibition of eating the flesh of pigs, dogs, cats, and so on. So also in some countries there is prohibition of eating the flesh of monkeys by pregnant women. We have to ask ourselves, however, if having these animals living with us is not a more common way of contracting diseases and of having parasites transmitted to us.

It is necessary to distinguish between traditions based on sound experience or on false or inadequate premises. To conclude, I shall repeat the advice I gave to my students, 'Consider yourselves as the pupils of the village community, have regard for teachings you do not understand, make efforts to find the explanations, the reasons for the traditions. It is only when you succeed in understanding that you might be bold enough to demythologize the prohibitions or other traditions which are held'.

REFERENCES

Castro, J. de (1952). *Geopolitique de la faim* (ed. Boyd Orr). Ouvrières, Paris.
Cépède, M. (1962). Demographie et developpement. *Cahiers de l'JSEA* (fevrier). Paris.
— (1970). Nutrition et sociologie. *Cahiers de Nutrition et diététique* (juin). Paris.
Dido, Fermin (1865). *Livre de Marco Polo.* Paris.
Lengellé, M. and Cépède, M. (1953). *Economic Alimentaire du globe,* Préface d'André Mayer, Gérvin, Paris.
Richet, C. and Mans, A. (1965). *La famine.* Paris.
Trémolières, J. (1969). Address to the International Congress of Nutrition, Prague.

3   Nutrition problems in the industrialized world

WILLIAM J. DARBY

The developing world and the industrialized world are but differing stages of history. Although marked contrasts exist between these regions there is a continuous spectrum of development through which country after country moves, some slowly, some more rapidly. Modern industrialization is a phenomenon of barely a century and a quarter; some industrialized countries have attained that stage only since the Second World War.

During the past 50 years I have observed the emergence of my home region, the Southern portion of the USA, from a rural, under-developed, economically impoverished area with a high prevalence of classical deficiency diseases, parasitic infestations, and infectious diseases of the young, into a prosperous industrialized, urbanized, agricultural region with no clinically detectable classical dietary deficiency diseases. In the 1920s and early 1930s the US Public Health Service reports from this region reached some 68 000 deaths annually and 4 to 10 times that number in morbidity from pellagra —there were mental institutions populated by pellagrins. Rickets, scurvy, hookworm anaemia and dwarfism, protein-calorie deficiency oedema and marasmus were commonly seen, the latter in infants and young children, especially during and following the period of 'summer diarrhoea'; megaloblastic anaemia of folic acid deficiency occurred among infants, macrocytic anaemia and sprue among adults (Hess 1920, 1929; Miller 1978; Minot, Dodd, Keller, and Frank 1940; Terris 1964; Washburn 1960; Woodruff and Peterson 1951). These conditions have disappeared and other health improvements have occurred—including as elsewhere in the US a great decline in incidence (and severity) of tuberculosis, poliomyelitis, syphilis, typhoid, and many other infectious diseases, and a continuing decrease in the infant death rate to its all-time low, and an increase in life expectancy to its all-time greatest.

THE PERSPECTIVE FROM THE VANTAGE POINT OF ATTAINMENT

I submit that much is to be gained by examining the relevant forces associated with or contributing to examples of nutritional and health improvements that occur with industrial development. In these experiences are significant lessons for many people who are at other bands in the spectrum of development, lessons that can improve nutritional health and minimize the nutritional risks inherent in sociocultural alterations accompanying economic and industrial development.

In 1971 W.R. Aykroyd considered how such an analysis of development in England could guide measures for solving problems of protein-calorie malnutrition today. The following passage was quoted by Aykroyd from a report on conditions in England in 1861 by Sir John Simon relating to nutrition of infants of factory workers:

Factory women soon return to labour after their confinement. . . .The mother's health suffers in consequence of this early return to labour. . .and the influence on the health and mortality of children is most baneful . . .care of their infants during their absence is entrusted either to young children, to hired girls, or perhaps more commonly to elderly women. . . .Pap, made of bread and water, and sweetened with sugar or treacle, is the sort of nourishment usually given during the mother's absence. . . . Illness is the natural consequence of this unnatural mode of feeding infants. . . .Children who are healthy at birth rapidly dwindle under this system of mismanagement, fall into bad health, and become uneasy, restless and fractious. . .

Abundant proof of the large mortality among children of female factory workers was obtained.

Examination of similar evidence in the United States during the period of 1880–1900 reveals that approximately half of the infants born died by five years of age and that scurvy, rickets, and other nutritional diseases were prevalent.

Bo Vahlquist wrote of Sweden (von Rosenstein 1976):

In . . . the mid-eighteenth century, as in all other countries at that time, the death roll among children was extremely high; 20 to 30% died in infancy and 50% were often lost before the age of five years. These are figures which today are found only in the most backward of the developing countries.

Aykroyd underscored the similarities of these earlier problems in countries now developed with those existing today in developing ones. He stated:

Whereas there may be a few discrepancies, it is reasonable to suppose that something like the complex of malnutrition and infection that we now call protein-calorie malnutrition [PCM] was prevalent in the affluent countries until recently, with disastrous effects on infant and child health. Clinical observations and vital statistics show that it has almost entirely disappeared from these countries. Its disappearance has been hastened by the establishment and development of maternal and child health services and centers (which began between 1900 and 1910), better housing and sanitation and higher levels of education accompanied by a general rise in living standards.

The most important factor has been improvement in infant and child feeding, associated with the introduction of safe milk, processed infant foods, mixtures based on cow's milk, and the education of mothers in hygienic feeding methods. Greater reliance on breast milk has played no part in reducing infant mortality in the affluent countries. . . . In fact, breast feeding has declined almost to the vanishing point during the last 40 to 50 years in most of these countries, a period that has seen a transformation in infant and child health.

Experience thus suggests that PCM can be eliminated in a few decades by the establishment of adequate maternal and child health services, rising standards of living, and hygienic artificial feeding. Examples of this can be found not only in highly developed countries in the temperate zone, but also in poor countries in the tropics, e.g. Barbados and Puerto Rico.

He concluded:

Experience in the affluent countries has shown that this complex [PCM] can be rapidly eliminated by efficient health services, rising standards of living, and hygienic artificial feeding. Greater reliance on breast feeding has played no part in its disappearance. The most promising method of attacking PCM in the developing countries is to promote the production and use of cheap feeding mixtures, based on plant foods that fulfill the infant's needs for calories, protein, and other nutrients.

Such is the perspective from a vantage point of realistic historical progress and human betterment through application of knowledge of the science of nutrition and medicine.

Elsewhere I reviewed briefly the experience in the United States (Darby 1976):

During the earlier development of industrialized food systems some deficiency states arose, but these do not occur in modern times because of the awareness of nutrition requirements and the nutritional quality of foods. The experience in perfecting scientifically-planned artificial infant feeding in the United States may be cited. During the later decades of the 19th century and early decades of the present one, protein deficiency, scurvy, rickets, and iron deficiency anemia were common among infants and young children because of the inadequacies of feeding regimens. The scientific design of the composition of infant formulas with attention to our 'newer knowledge of nutrition,' combined with hygienic measures in the preparation of food and water and the wide availability of suitable foods for babies eliminated these diseases as scourges. These developments have been accompanied by the remarkable reduction in morbidity and mortality rates among infants and the under five year old group.

From such a vantage point of accomplished nutritional benefits, perspectives on many problems may be obtained. The potential for practical, rapid alleviation of a variety of preventable deficiency states through enrichment and fortification has been documented (WHO 1960)—these include iodine-deficiency goitre, pellagra, beriberi, ariboflavinosis, vitamin-A deficiency, rickets, nutritional anaemias (iron or folate deficiency or both), and others. General guidelines have been proposed for the beneficial utilization of industrially produced nutrients, as well as for using specific nutrients such as vitamin A and iron (Darby and Hambraeus 1975). Initiation of such a programme is contingent upon several factors, one of which is identifying a suitable, generally consumed, centrally processed food to serve as the vehicle for controllable economical addition of the nutrient(s). The nutrients must be stable in the foodstuff as distributed and used. Success is dependent upon acceptability of food to the consumer and some understanding of its value. Proper nutrition education is essential.

SOME CORRELATES OF NUTRITION AND AFFLUENT LIFE-STYLES

Other health changes, the so-called diseases of the affluent society, may accompany industrialization; but these are not attributable to alteration in nutrient value of individual foods. They reflect the profound differences in life-styles between the rural non-industrialized society and the urbanized industrial complex and also the increased survival time and longevity resulting from scientific development. None of these diseases, however, is a stranger to societies that are scientifically untouched. Modern application of scientific knowledge of the health and food sciences and proper recognition of nutritional needs can reduce the toll from these diseases.

What important basic influences in the industrially developed community bear on nutriture and directly or indirectly on these diseases? Time will not allow identification and discussion of all, but let us consider a few in order to focus more effectively our educational efforts.

1. Nutritional drain or excessive demands for nutrients are minimal because:
   (a) parasitic and infectious diseases are eliminated or controlled;
   (b) labour-intensive occupations are few and labour-saving devices reduce energy expenditure of both men and women;
   (c) environmental temperatures are controlled and there are minimal expenditures for heat regulation; and
   (d) there are few pregnancies per woman and lactation is abbreviated.

2. Food is readily available, much of it of high nutrient (including caloric) density and periods of food shortages and seasonal variations in supply are eliminated.

3. The variety of foodstuffs readily available is wide and includes cereals, tubers, vegetables, fruits, animal products of all categories (meat, milk, cheese and dairy products, poultry, eggs, fish and seafoods), condiments, alcoholic and non-alcoholic beverages, oils and fats, specialty foods, and sweets.

4. Few foods are grown or harvested by the consumer himself, a decreasing number are prepared by him, and many meals are served in predetermined portions.

5. The ready availability of food coupled with reduced physiological need renders facile excessive caloric consumption to the point of obesity, a risk factor in:
(a) late onset diabetes,
(b) some cardiovascular disease, and
(c) a variety of somewhat less serious causes of morbidity.

6. Prolonged life span results in an aging population with accumulation of diseases attendant to later life—diabetes, cardiovascular-renal diseases, cancer, osteoporosis, emphysema, and senility itself.

Two important nutritional characteristics of our society are:

1. Except for the unusual culturally or socio-economically isolated subculture or for medically conditioned states, (e.g. malabsorption, long-term nutritional maintenance by non-oral route, chronic alcoholism, chronic blood loss, etc.) classical deficiency diseases are exceedingly rare.

2. Low energy expenditure and ready access to an abundance of food facilitates excessive intake and enhances the potential for developing obesity with its associated health risks. Increased life span allows development of diseases attendant to later years of life.

IMPLICATIONS OF LIMITED CALORIC REQUIREMENT FOR
TYPE OF DIET

Are there other implications of the relatively low dietary energy requirements of man in the industrialized society? An energy intake of 3000 to 4000 calories supplied by a variety of food groups will likely supply adequate quantities of all essential nutrients even if some foods are of limited nutrient density. A usual mixed diet in Scandinavia, Britain, or North America provides 6 mg or less of iron per 1000 calories daily; a woman ingesting 1800 or 2000 calories per day therefore obtains 10–12 mg of dietary iron. This amount is insufficient to meet current standards of allowances (*Recommended dietary allowances* 1974) for women, especially during pregnancy and lactation (Wretlind 1968). Its adequacy may be further compromised if the dietary composition is not such as to favour iron absorption, i.e. if it is devoid or low in meat or high in bulk or phytate.

The nutrient density (Hansen 1973), e.g. the ratio of quantity of other essential nutrients to energy content of the diet, must be higher for a low calorie intake than for a high calorie diet.

The composition of the food intake in industrialized areas varies but is in the range of some 12–15 per cent of calories from protein, 35–45 per cent from fat, and the remainder from carbohydrate and alcohol. Carbohydrate is supplied as starches, sugars, dextrans, sugar alcohols, etc. In recent years, the carbohydrate supply per capita in the United States has remained essentially stationary (Sipple and McNutt 1974); the sugar (sucrose) supply per capita likewise has remained essentially constant in the United States and Europe. Indeed, there is a tendency for sugar 'consumption' to level at a little over 100 lb per capita per year. In countries where it has significantly exceeded this level, it tends to decrease to it. In the US sugar consumption per capita has held at approximately 100–10 lb per year since the 1920s. Consumption of starch has decreased somewhat, the difference being replaced by other sugars, syrups, and carbohydrate derivatives (Sipple and McNutt 1974).

The contributions of alcoholic beverages to the caloric intake of individuals (Darby, Gastineau, and Turner, in press) is less well documented than are the data for other foodstuffs. For many adults, alcoholic beverages constitute 5–15 per cent of their caloric intake; for some it may be as great as 40–50 per cent.

The inborn taste for sweetness has been well documented; (Sipple and McNutt 1974) history confirms that man will not forgo satisfying that sense. Similarly, affluent societies will not forgo the pleasures of alcoholic beverages except under the greatest duress.

The obvious implications of these facts for the diet of the affluent are often missed by those in nutrition education and planning who fail to or refuse to view the broad picture as it is displayed.

Caloric needs determine the limits of food that can healthily be ingested. These needs are small because of the life-style of the affluent. In order to maintain desirable protective levels of nutrients in the diet consistent with the acceptable food habits of society, some 40–50 per cent of the total diet must consist of high-nutrient density foodstuffs supplying needed quantities of the essential nutrients: amino acids, vitamins, minerals, and trace elements. This means that 40–60 per cent of the energy value of the diet must be derived from high nutrient density foodstuffs: products such as meat, milk, eggs, cheese, vegetables, fruits, and cereals. In order further to maintain nutrient density of the diet, selected enhancement of the nutrient content of some foodstuffs, such as cereals, is desirable (Darby and Hambraeus 1975). Newly formulated foodstuffs, such as food analogues, are nutritionally designed and consideration should be given to increasing selected nutrients in low nutrient density foodstuffs (Darby and Hambraeus 1975).

Positive, innovative educational and motivational efforts should be directed toward the selection and use of high nutrient density foods in sufficient amounts and with sufficient regularity to provide a nutritious diet within acceptable caloric limits.

SOME CHALLENGES TO NUTRITION EDUCATION

Nutrition education should not be divorced from educational motivation toward altering living patterns to increase the physical fitness and caloric expenditure of the sedentary adult within the industrialized society.

The ubiquitous modes of free communication—the press, print media generally, radio, and television—offer unprecedented educational opportunities. The challenge here is to evolve effective, economically feasible means of utilizing the media. For true educational programmes to gain access to the costly media, their appeal must be competitive with sensational entertainment. The nutritional quack or faddist more successfully competes with entertainers than does the responsible nutrition scientist and educator. The dramatic uninhibited claims of the faddist or quack contrast to the factual caution of the scientist. Programme planners and media personnel therefore spotlight the dramatic to gain audience appeal. I do not have time to elaborate on the enormous amount of 'hogwash' from nutrition quacks, faddists, and misdirected, sometimes self-serving scientists that reaches the public through these media channels (*Nutrition misinformation and food faddism* 1974), but it remains a major challenge to us as educators.

I regard this Conference as a giant step forward in advancing nutrition knowledge and its effective application for improving the health and welfare of mankind—the stated objective of the Nutrition Foundation.

The complexity of our task in developed countries is succinctly illustrated in the summary on nutrition education prepared by the National Nutrition Consortium in its *Guidelines for a National Nutrition Policy* (1974):

Nutrition information should be incorporated into all levels of formal education.

a. In schools: Nutrition should be a basic curriculum requirement in all elementary schools and high schools. The school lunch program should be used to assist in nutrition education through correlation with teaching in the classroom.
   All teachers should receive training in nutrition.
   Courses in nutrition should be available in colleges and universities.

b. Training of nutrition professionals and para-professionals, physicians, diet-itians, public health nutritionists, dentists, nurses, veterinarians, social workers, physical educators should have high priority. Both undergraduate and post-graduate training is needed as well as continuing education.

Medical schools should be encouraged to establish faculty and resources for teaching nutrition in clinical as well as preclinical departments and nutrition training and services should be promoted in hospitals and clinics.

The Land Grant Universities (schools of agriculture) should continue and expand training in the areas of food and nutrition.

c. Sound nutrition information for the general public should be carried out through all components of the communications media, including federal, state and local departments of education, Cooperative State Extension Services, colleges and universities, community agencies, industry and the mass media.

Food labeling and food advertising can contribute significantly to nutrition knowledge. Labeling and advertising regulations should require presentation of truthful nutrition information in all instances where nutritional claims are made.

Nutrition education can be incorporated in such programs as the food stamp program and in supplementary feeding programs.

We in the United States have not attained these goals despite much recent progress. I hope that the Conference will have helped accelerate the progress toward such national goals in all nations represented.

REFERENCES

Aykroyd, W.R. (1971). Nutrition and mortality in infancy and early childhood: past and present relationships. *Am. J. Clin. Nutr.* 24, 480–7.

Darby, W.J. (1976). Benefit-risk decision-making and food safety. Chapter in *Food, man and society*. Plenum, New York.

—— and Hambraeus, L. (1975). Proposed nutritional guidelines for utilization of industrially produced nutrients. *Näringsforskning, Arg.* 19, 113–20.

See also: *Guidelines for the eradication of vitamin A deficiency and xerophthal-mia* (1976). Report of the International Vitamin A Consultative Group (IVACG), The Nutrition Foundation, New York and Washington, D.C.

Guidelines for the eradication of iron deficiency anemia (1977). Report of the International Nutritional Anemia Consultative Group (INACG), The Nutrition Foundation, New York and Washington, D.C.

Guidelines for a national nutrition policy (1974). National Nutrition Con-sortium, Inc. *Nutr. Rev.* 32, (5).

—— Gastineau, C.F., and Turner, T.B. *Fermented Food Beverages in Nutrition*, Academic Press, New York. (In press).

Hansen, R.G. (1973). An index of food quality. *Nutr. Rev.* 31(1).

Hess, A.F. (1920). *Scurvy past and present.* Lippincott Co., Philadelphia.

—— (1929). *Rickets, including osteomalacia and tetany.* Lea and Febiger, Philadelphia.

Inadequate Diets and Nutritional Deficiencies in the United States, (1943) Bulletin of the National Research Council, No. 109, National Research Council, National Academy of Sciences, Washington, DC, November.

Miller, D.F. (1978) Pellagra deaths in the United States. *Am. J. Clin. Nutr.* 31, (4).

Minot, A.S., Dodd, K., Keller, M., and Frank, H. (1940) Survey of the state of nutrition with respect to vitamin C in Southern pediatric clinics. *J. Pediat.* **16**, 717–28.

Nutrition misinformation and food faddism (1974). A special supplement, *Nutr. Rev.* **32**, Supplement No. 1 (July).

See also: Blix, G. (Ed.) (1970). *Food cultism and nutrition quackery.* The Swedish Nutrition Foundation, Uppsala.

Barrett, S. and Knight, G. (Ed.) (1976). *The health robbers.* George F. Stickley Co., Philadelphia.

Recommended dietary allowances. (1974). Eighth edition. Food and Nutrition Board, National Research Council, National Academy of Sciences, Washington, DC.

Rosenstein, N.R. von (1976) *The diseases of children and their remedies.* Nutrition Foundation Reprint, Johnson Reprint Corporation, New York (1977).

Sipple, H.L. and McNutt, K.W. (Eds.) (1974). *Sugars in nutrition.* Academic Press, New York.

Terris, M. (Ed.) (1964). *Goldberger on pellagra,* Louisiana State University Press, Baton Rouge, Louisiana.

Washburn, B.E. (1960) *As I recall: The hookworm campaign initiated by the Rockefeller Sanitary Commission and the Rockefeller Foundation in the Southern U.S. and tropical America.* Office of Publications, Rockefeller Foundation, New York.

Weiffenbach, J.M. *Taste and Development: The Genesis of Sweet Preference,* DHEW Publication No. (NIH) 77-1068, U.S. Department of Health, Education and Welfare, Public Health Service, National Institutes of Health, Bethesda, Maryland, 1977.

Woodruff, C.W. and Peterson, J.C. (1951). *Postgrad. Med.* **10**, 189.

See also: Quelzer, W.W. and Ogden, F.N. (1946). *Am. J. Dis. Child.* **71**, 211.

Youmans, J.B. *et al.* (1942, 1943) Nutrition surveys in Middle Tennessee. *Am. J. Publ. Health* **32**, 1371 (1942), **33**, 58, 955 (1943).

Hanes, F. (1946). Sprue. In *Tice's practice of Medicine.* W.F. Pryor Co., Inc., Hagerstown, Md.

World Health Organization Monograph Series, No. 44, Geneva (1960).

See also: *Iodine nutriture in the United States.* Summary of a Conference, October 31, 1970, Food and Nutrition Board, National Academy of Sciences, Washington, DC.

Enrichment of flour and bread—a history of the movement. Bulletin of the National Research Council, No. 110, National Research Council, National Academy of Sciences, Washington, DC, November (1944).

Cereal enrichment in perspective, 1958. Food and Nutrition Board, National Research Council, National Academy of Sciences, Washington, DC.

Proposed fortification policy for cereal-grain products. Food and Nutrition Board, National Research Council, National Academy of Sciences, Washington, DC. (1974).

Technology of fortification of foods. Food and Nutrition Board, National Research Council, National Academy of Sciences, Washington, DC. (1975).

Wretlind, A. (1968). The supply of food iron. Chapter in *Occurence, causes and prevention of nutrition anemias* (Ed. G. Blix). The Swedish Nutrition Foundation, Uppsala.

4 Nutritional problems in developing countries

C. GOPALAN

The poor countries of Asia, Africa, and Latin America, which are often euphemistically referred to as the developing world, today account for nearly 75 per cent of the world's population. Some of the striking differences between these poor developing countries, on the one hand, and the affluent technologically developed countries on the other need to be highlighted since they have an important bearing on the nutrition problem. I referred to these on an earlier occasion, but it will be appropriate to recall them here.

Two contrasting food chains are in evidence in these two groups of countries. The poor countries of the developing world, depend on the plant-to-man food chain; while the affluent countries of Europe and North America depend on the plant–animal–man food chain. Thus, out of the average consumption of food grains per capita of about one tonne per year in the affluent countries, only about 70 kg are consumed directly, while the remaining 930 kg are used as animal food to raise meat, milk, and eggs for human consumption. In contrast, the consumption of grain per capita per year in the developing countries is about 190 kg most of which is directly consumed. Thus, the implications of food-grain shortage are totally different as between a country like, say, India and a country like the USSR. In one case, food-grain shortage may mean starvation, while, in the other, it may just mean a reduction in the current high levels of intake of animal protein. The daily intake of protein in the diet of adults of developing countries is of the order of 50 g, a level which is adequate to meet the protein needs, and the protein is largely derived from vegetable sources. As against this, the daily intake of proein in the diet of adults of many affluent countries exceeds 100 g daily, and the protein is largely derived from animal sources, an intake which is clearly far in excess of physiological needs.

There are also important differences in the pattern of food production as between the developing and developed countries. In the affluent countries, with increasing mechanization, the prevailing trend is for larger and larger farms to be managed by fewer cultivators. On the other hand, in many poor countries, smaller and smaller farms have to be cultivated by the same or even larger number of farmers. The highly mechanized, capital-intensive, and labour-saving technology of the affluent countries is just not feasible in the developing countries. Also, agricultural operations in affluent countries are based on high-consumption of energy derived from non-renewable resources of the earth. Thus while about 280 kcal of energy are needed in countries like India and Indonesia to produce 1 kg of rice protein, as much as 2860 kcal are needed to produce 1 kg of wheat protein and over 65 000 kcal to produce 1 kg of beef protein in the United States. While 95 per cent of the energy input in the USA in 1970 came from oil, gas, and coal, in the same year non-commercial fuels like cow-dung, firewood, and wastes provided 60 per cent of India's fuel needs. If the developing world were to imitate the current technology of affluent countries for food production, the world's oil wells would run dry in a decade. The great challenge that faces the developing world, then, is continuously to increase the productivity of land using a labour-intensive technology with minimal dependence on non-renewable sources of energy.

Let me next turn to a major determinant of nutritional status, namely the pattern of population growth. Many developing countries have populations expanding at the rate of 2.5–3.5 per cent per year. In Europe, on the other hand, the rate is around 0.5 per cent and is practically at zero in a number of countries. Infant and child mortality in most affluent countries is already so low that there is not much scope for further improvement. On the other hand, in many developing countries death rates, which are still high, may be expected to show a continuing decline over the next few decades. As a result of these contrasting trends, a preponderant proportion of the increase of world population in the next two decades will be accounted for by increase in the population of developing countries. It may be computed that the world population, which stood at around 3600 million in 1970, may exceed 6600 million by AD 2000 and nearly 90 per cent of this increase will be accounted for by increase in the populations of Africa, Asia, and Latin America. Such a population increase may be expected to greatly accentuate pressure on the already severely strained facilities for health care, food, housing, and education in these countries.

The process of economic polarization of the world into the affluent 'haves' and poor 'have-nots' continues on its relentless course. Any hope that the statesmen of the world will evolve a new ethos in international relationships which will ensure the judicious exploitation and husbanding of the world's resources for the maximal benefit of all mankind will not be justified by the hard realities of the present-day world. To the developing world, the nutritional problem, which is already formidable, will become a challenge of growing magnitude in the next few decades. While the nutrition problem is already at the centre of the public-health stage in these countries, all indications point to a further aggravation of the problem in the coming decades. The prospects of our being able to control some of the major infectious diseases in the developing countries in the coming decades would appear to be reasonably bright. On the other hand, futuristic projections of trends in population growth and food production present a rather grim picture. Malnutrition will thus emerge as the major health problem of the developing world in the next few decades.

In the ultimate analysis, undernutrition is but one manifestation of the 'poverty syndrome' afflicting large segments of the populations of the developing countries. The other attributes of the 'poverty syndrome' are unemployment or underemployment, poor sanitation, poor housing and clothing, and a low level of literacy. The synergistic relationship between undernutrition and infection generating a vicious cycle leading to accelerating deterioration of health is now well known. The low level of literacy plays an important contributory role; even the limited food resources and health facilities available are often not effectively utilized to maximal advantage; and faulty dietary and living habits arising from ignorance tend to aggravate the situation.

Under these circumstances, in the long run, the nutritional uplift of these poor population groups can come about only as part and parcel of overall socio-economic development, and not just through isolated health programmes or *ad hoc* nutrition programmes. However, economic development and overall increase in GNP need not necessarily be reflected in eradication of poverty and improvement in nutrition, unless such economic development is accompanied by social and distributive justice. Unfortunately in many developing countries where undernutrition is a serious problem glaring socio-economic disparities persist. Thus, according to some estimates nearly 30 per cent of the population of some developing countries live below the 'poverty line', meaning that even if this population group expend 90 per cent of their total income on food, they will still not be able to afford even the least-cost adequate balanced diet. Under the circumstances, mere increase in food production in the country will not solve the problem of undernutrition unless the purchasing power of the poor segments is raised to levels at which they can buy the foods they need. On the other hand, a strategy of development in these developing countries, which only serves to make the rich even richer will only widen social disparities, aggravate deprivation among the poor, and prove counter-productive. What the developing countries should opt for instead is a strategy of development which will involve the bulk of the people in productive endeavour and thus raise their income levels and socio-economic status. All programmes of socio-economic development based on such a strategy, which contribute to the eradication of poverty, will facilitate the elimination of undernutrition and are thus to be welcomed and encouraged from the nutritional point of view.

While it is thus true that undernutrition in the developing countries today is a part of the general poverty syndrome and can therefore be eradicated in the long run, only through socio-economic development can a great deal be done to mitigate undernutrition in these countries even in the prevailing socio-economic situation. There are many 'natural experiments' which will support this conclusion. In many poor communities subsisting on uniformly inadequate diets only a relatively small proportion of children suffer from severe grades of malnutrition; a high proportion suffer from moderate grades of malnutrition, and a very small percentage from just marginal malnutrition. These differences in the grades of malnutrition cannot be explained on the basis of differences in income levels, living conditions, or socio-economic status. A study carried out by the National Institute of Nutrition, Hyderabad, India, a few years ago showed that in poor communities living on uniform inadequate diets, it was the children of mothers who were particularly ignorant and lacking in resourcefulness and motivation that developed kwashiorkor. A large proportion of poor children even in these very poor communities escaped from serious forms of undernutrition, presumably because the poor mothers in these cases were able to use their meagre resources in the matter of food or public-health services to maximal advantage. This point can be even more convincingly illustrated through data available from two states of the Indian Union namely Kerala in the extreme south and Uttar Pradesh in the north. According to the latest available figures, the infant mortality rate in Kerala is around 55 per thousand as against 161 per thousand in Uttar Pradesh. The neonatal mortality (mortality in infants under one month of age) is 33 per thousand in Kerala as against 72 per thousand in Uttar Pradesh. Life expectancy at birth is 64 years in Kerala and 55 in Uttar Pradesh. Deaths of children under 5 years account for 19 per cent of all deaths in Kerala and 35 per cent in Uttar Pradesh.

These differences cannot be explained on the basis of socio-economic differences or food availability per capita because with respect to these Kerala is no better than Uttar Pradesh. What perhaps is significant is that the literacy rate in Kerala is 67 per cent in males and nearly 54 per cent in females as against 31 per cent and 11 per cent respectively in Uttar Pradesh. Of all children between 11 to 14 years, 75 per cent are in schools in Kerala as against 28 per cent in Uttar Pradesh. I believe that the differences between Kerala and Uttar Pradesh can be largely if not wholly explained on the basis of this striking difference in the female literacy ratio, and are a convincing indication of the crucial role of education. This observation is of practical importance, as this is a comparison not between two different countries with entirely different socio-economic and cultural conditions but between two parts of the same country. If the rest of India can be moved to the Kerala end of the public health and nutrition spectrum within the next two decades, we would have achieved a great deal.

In poor socio-economic groups, it is especially important to ensure that locally available inexpensive foods are used to maximal advantage and in this context nutrition education acquires added importance. For example with respect to the problem of protein calorie malnutrition, which is widespread, it is now generally recognized that judicious combinations of locally available inexpensive vegetable foods can go a long way in mitigating the problem. Poor countries need not wait for specially processed protein-rich foods and concentrates. We know from all available evidence that if calorie needs are satisfied through such relatively inexpensive foods as cereals and legumes, the protein needs are also largely met. This should offer hope to poor communities and invests nutrition education programmes among these communities with crucial significance. Recipes for weaning foods based on such locally available inexpensive foods, capable of preparation at the home or village level, offer promise of mitigation, if not of eradication, of the problem of protein calorie malnutrition.

With respect to other widespread problems of undernutrition such as vitamin-A deficiency and anaemia, modern technology is now able to provide answers which are capable of application even in the current socio-economic context of the developing countries. The demonstration that massive doses of vitamin A given orally once in six months can mitigate the problem of vitamin-A deficiency among young children, places in the hands of nutrition workers a practical, if not an ideal, tool with which to combat the problem of vitamin-A deficiency for immediate use. The possibilities of our being able to prevent iron-deficiency anaemia through fortification with iron of foods like common salt have now become bright;

large-scale application of this technology should help to control iron-deficiency anaemia which at present is extremely widespread not only among pregnant women but also among children in many developing countries subsisting on cereal staples rich in phytate, which interferes with iron absorption.

Apart from nutritional deficiency diseases, recent studies indicate that there are several diseases occurring among the poor which are attributable to the contamination of food with either 'natural' or other toxins arising from poor storage conditions. Thus the food available to these poor communities is not only inadequate, but is often unwholesome as well. I can provide three examples of such diseases. It has been shown by the National Institute of Nutrition, Hyderabad, that the problem of neurolathyrism, which afflicts considerable sections of the poor population in central India and which is associated with excessive consumption of the pulse *Lathyrus sativus*, can be prevented through the application of the simple process of parboiling the pulse. This helps to eliminate the toxic factor BOAA (β-(N)-oxalyl amino alanine) present in the pulse which is responsible for the neurological damage. Again it has been demonstrated that the occurrence of hepatic damage—veno-occlusive disease—among the millet eaters in central India is attributable to the admixture of the millet seeds with the seeds of *Crotalaria*, the latter containing toxic alkaloids. The disorder can be completely prevented by quite simply sieving out the toxic weeds—a task easily performed by the rural housewife in her own home.

The occurrence of some epidemic outbreaks of liver disease in India has now shown to be related to the consumption of food grains contaminated by the fungus *Aspergillus flavus*. The infection arises from the storage of food grains under moist conditions. Simple improvements in food-storage practices can completely eliminate this situation.

The important point, however, is that the application of even these relatively simple technologies among poor communities calls for community acceptance and motivation. A sustained programme of nutrition education is an essential prerequisite for the success of these measures. In the absence of such a programme of nutrition education for the communities, many of these programmes to control disease have languished. Many worthwhile nutrition intervention programmes among poor communities have not made much headway since the importance of the educational component has on the whole not been appreciated.

In many developing countries, vast amounts of money have been expended—and are still being expended—on supplementary feeding programmes and school-lunch programmes. These programmes can be a most valuable means of nutrition education; in fact nutrition education is often stated to be a major objective of these programmes. In actual practice, however, it is the mechanics of the feeding operation that takes up all the attention in these programmes and the objective of nutrition education is completely lost. It is no wonder then that these programmes, in spite of impressive investments, have often failed to leave any lasting impact on the poor communities. Poor rural mothers, instead of being enlisted as active participants in these programmes, are often bypassed altogether as they are considered to be potential hurdles and obstacles to the programmes. Experience with agricultural extension programmes in many developing countries has shown that the poor illiterate peasant in rural areas is by no means unintelligent; he is quite willing to accept and adopt any new technology provided its practical value is convincingly demonstrated to him. Unfortunately in the field of health and nutrition we have largely failed to do this.

It is now generally recognized that the most rewarding strategy in combating undernutrition in many developing countries will be an integrated programme which will include the following mutually reinforcing components: (1) improvement of environmental sanitation; (2) immunization; (3) family planning; (4) specific nutrition services; and (5) health education. Isolated nutrition programmes divorced from the other components of the package may prove ineffective and wasteful. A nutrition-education programme must also be part of a wider programme of community education and development and must be tailored to meet the special needs of the community and to promote the acceptance and implementation of other developmental measures.

The delivery of such a composite package of integrated programmes, calls for the existence of an infrastructure of institutional facilities and trained manpower that will enable the health and welfare agencies to *reach* the poor communities. Unfortunately this does not appear to be the case in several developing countries and a radical reorientation of the public-health infrastructure would seem necessary. More than 75 per cent of the inputs in the field of public health in many developing countries are now deployed for the benefit of less than 20 per cent of the population.

The bulk of the rural poor in the developing countries do not often have the benefit of even basic minimal health care. The outreach of Maternal and Child Health (MCH) and health centres is often so inadequate that only a small segment of the total population at risk is reached by these services. Under these circumstances, perhaps, the most outstanding contribution to health and nutrition in many developing countries would be the institution of a new strategy which will promote a better outreach of health services to the rural poor. Even if adequate outreach of the health services is achieved, it will still be necessary to ensure that nutrition receives adequate emphasis in the health and welfare programmes. The nutrition component in the package of health and welfare services has to be clearly defined and delineated and the personnel engaged in the delivery of these services adequately trained and oriented.

Several developing countries are now attempting to increase the outreach of their basic health services through the identification and training of community-level workers. These workers belong to the village and are largely drawn from the poor socio-economic group. It is proposed that they should be given training for a short duration in basic skills related to the delivery of health care so that they may at least provide the first order of health service to the communities and help in 'referring' more serious ailments to health centres managed by doctors. It is extremely important that in the training of these community-level workers nutrition should find adequate emphasis. If this does not happen, there is the real danger that in the face of competing claims of other important health activities like immunization and family planning, nutrition may well be relegated to the background. The important challenge to nutrition workers is to ensure that a realistic nutrition component is built into the training of the village-level functionaries who are going to be in constant touch with the poor communities. The precise content of the nutrition component in the overall composite package of health services must be carefully tailored and designed to suit the special needs of the communities concerned and must also be realistic enough to be capable of implementation within the financial, institutional, and manpower constraints under which community programmes in poor countries have to labour. It is to be hoped that nutrition workers in developing countries will face up to this difficult challenge.

5 Changing concepts of healthy diets in prosperous communities

A.S. TRUSWELL

There was an outstanding system of nutrition education organized by the Ministry of Food in Britain during the Second World War. Today we can only admire the writing and artwork and envy the enthusiastic public response. The messages are no longer really applicable.

The basic concepts of nutrition education have changed radically in the last 25 years. The two major impacts were the rediscovery and general recognition of kwashiorkor in developing countries (Brock and Autret 1952), and the dietary fat hypothesis of coronary heart disease in affluent countries (Keys 1952). As faster travel has made the world seem to contract, nutritional knowledge has grown in the developing countries, initially because of expatriates like Aykroyd and Passmore in India; Waterlow in Jamaica; Scrimshaw in Guatemala; Cicely Williams and Aylward in Ghana; Trowell, McCance, and Whitehead in Uganda; French and Swedish workers elsewhere in Africa; Dutch workers in New Guinea; Darby and colleagues in the Middle East. They responded to the challenge and set up special nutrition research units. In many areas the nutritional state has improved.

But in turn the industrial, temperate-latitude countries have learnt important lessons from developing countries. You don't have to consume milk to grow normally (indeed many are actually intolerant of large quantities) or consume meat for strength—cereals and other staples supply important amounts of protein and not only starch; and the fibrous parts of plant foods may be beneficial for health (Burkitt 1973; Trowell 1972). Some communities have much lower plasma cholesterols than in those eating a northern European type of diet and rarely experience coronary heart disease; nor are obesity in middle age or constipation inevitable. They are associated with the North American/European way of life, including the diet.

There is a fundamental difference between ideas of how to improve diets in developing and prosperous communities. In developing countries the object is to reduce malnutrition, which is often acute and clinically manifest. You can see the effects of your advice or provision of food in a short time in individuals. Better infant and child feeding, if successfully implemented, will be followed more or less promptly by less protein-energy malnutrition; with better weights and heights and less illness in the community; iodization of salt should be followed in a year or two by less goitre, and so on. But in prosperous countries (some of which form minorities in developing countries) most of the current dietary recommendations are based on epidemiology rather than acute paediatric or medical experience. Diet is often only one of a complex of factors related, after many years exposure, to an increased probability (not certainty) of one or more chronic diseases. Modifying the diet will not usually have effects which convince the patient or members of the public or even some health professionals. Nutrition educators should never forget the apostle 'Doubting Thomas'. Two notable exceptions, ways in which a change of diet produces rapid physical change, are weight loss on reducing diets for obesity and alleviation of constipation with wheat fibre and some fruits. Even here most of us are only partially successful in managing obesity. To take extra fibre in the diet is no hardship and the reproducible rapid effect which everyone can observe privately for himself may explain the great public enthusiasm for the benefits of dietary fibre which has overtaken the pace of scientific research in this field.

In 1968 (*Var föda* 1963; Keys 1968), nutrition and health authorities in three Scandinavian countries made recommendations for improving the diets of ordinary people in Sweden, Norway, and Finland in order to prevent or reduce several chronic diseases while minimizing the remaining forms of malnutrition. These were:

less total calories for many people;

less total fat, reduced from 40 per cent to about 30 per cent of energy of this total fat, the proportion of saturated fat should be reduced and of polyunsaturated fat increased;

consumption of sugar and sugar-rich products should be reduced; and consumption of vegetables, fruit, potatoes, skimmed milk, fish, lean meat, and cereal products should be increased.

This is general advice, aimed at preventing several chronic diseases— dental caries, obesity (with all its complications), coronary heart disease, constipation and diverticulosis, etc.—and also to prevent malnutrition by advising reduction of foods low in essential nutrients, and which supply empty calories.

In several other countries authoritative bodies have made recommendations in the last 10 years about modification of diet and other habits to try and delay or prevent coronary heart disease. To date, 18 such expert committees have published advice in the last 9 years. As well as the Scandinavian countries, recommendations have been made in the USA (6 reports), Australia (2), New Zealand (2), Britain (2), The Netherlands, West Germany, and Canada.

But these have all concentrated on one disease; they are not general recommendations.

In February, this year the United States Senate's Select Committee on Nutrition and Human Needs published *Dietary goals for the United States* (Staff of the Select Committee on Nutrition and Human Needs, United States Senate 1977; *Lancet* 1977). They resemble the earlier Scandinavian recommendations in several items and are for general health.

(1) increase complex carbohydrate consumption—vegetables and fruit (preferably lightly or not processed) and cereals (preferably not refined);
(2) reduce total fat consumption to 30 per cent of energy;
(3) within the reduced total fat (a) reduce the proportion of saturated and (b) increase the proportion of polyunsaturated fat;
(4) reduce dietary cholesterol;
(5) reduce refined-sugar consumption;
(6) reduce salt (NaCl) consumption (a) for babies (b) in adults.

I considered these goals in a symposium held by the Nutrition Society recently (Truswell 1977) and concluded that goals 1, 2, 3a, 5, and 6a already had wide support in Britain—or in some cases appear to be government policy—but 3b was the subject of controversy while there was small acceptance of 4 or enthusiasm for 6b at present.

I suggested that the American goals could be made more comprehensive by adding another seven, all of which have been authoratively proposed or supported in this country:

(7) steps against obesity;*
(8) encouragement of breast-feeding in infants;
(9) reduction of unnecessary food additives;
(10) no further increase in alcohol consumption;
(11) provision of drinking water with optimal fluoride concentration;
(12) measures to reduce iron deficiency; and
(13) measures to prevent rickets and osteomalacia.

The resulting list of thirteen recommendations is hybrid (some are about foods, other about nutritional disorders). The thirteenth goal is a special British problem. Each country is likely to have its special nutritional problem: it might even be prevention of an infectious disease transmitted in the food. Most of the other goals could well be considered in many prosperous communities—including the upper socio-economic classes of rapidly developing countries.

The order in which I have put these 13 goals is thematic and arbitrary. People could vote on a rearrangement in order of priority.

*In a second edition of the US *Dietary goals*, published in November 1977 an additional goal of preventing obesity has been added by Senator George McGovern's Committee.

Dietary goals like these are very different from the 3 food groups used in Britain during the Second World War or the 'basic 7' (1943) or 'basic 4' (1954) used in the USA (Hertzler and Anderson 1974) and other food groups for public education in nutrition (Ahlström and Räsänen 1973). The food groups have four important weaknesses. (a) They ignore the staple which provides a mixture of nutrients. It is misleading, for example, to teach children and the adult public that bread in northern Europe is only an energy food; it provides important proportions of protein, thiamin, fibre, etc. Nor are potatoes pure energy food. In northern Europe they often provide more vitamin C than any other food. (b) They all seem to include a separate group for foods providing calcium. This is quite illogical because dietary deficiency of calcium is hardly established by nutritional scientists as a reality while iron deficiency is widespread, but there is no separate group of foods to provide iron. (c) They tell the public nothing about preventing dental caries, obesity, hypertension, coronary heart disease, constipation, etc., the major nutritional disorders of our society and time. It is far better nutrition education to emphasize the harm to the teeth from much chewing of sticky sweets and to press for fluoridation of drinking water than to teach the public about providing a source of calcium each day. (d) There are too many sets of food groups. The public and even professors of nutrition get confused. In the fascinating exhibition of nutrition education posters at the Conference the section for one country, Great Britain, shows no fewer than 6 different sets of food groups in a small space, ranging from 3 or 4 up to 10 groups. Part of the reason for this is that food manufacturers obligingly provide posters and booklets about food groups for nutritionists. Who can blame the dairy industry, for example, for having a special group for good sources of calcium.

There are serious difficulties too in using recommended intakes, and hence nutrition labelling, as the main basis for nutrition education of the public. These put too much emphasis on micronutrients—riboflavin, niacin etc.—as against the major sources of energy. They give no advice about the ratio of fat, carbohydrate, and protein, or on the type of fat or carbohydrate or of fibre. Different countries have from 8 to 20 nutrients in their main table of recommended intakes and do not always include critical ones (Truswell 1976).

Nutrients vary in biological availability as they occur in foods. Some scientists think that there should be two levels of recommended intakes, a low level for assessment of food-intake data and a higher level for advice to the public and caterers (Wretlind 1977).

The new dietary goals assume the typical food pattern of a community and recommend which items should be decreased and which increased. Without the latter, advice is not practical. *Foods* rather than nutrients are now the currency. There is more to nutrition than providing the nutrients. These have to be balanced, but so do the potentially toxic compounds in all foods (natural, accidental, or artificial). And the packing, the 'dietary fibre' (which differs too between foods) is not physiologically inert.

Yet there is a relativity of food patterns: even in a single country the patterns differ between minorities; for example Asians living in Britain; groups with unconventional social values, vegetarians, vegans, and adherents of an alternative society. The more complex the country, the more difficult it is to cater for the various minorities by mass media. There are still minor but not insignificant differences in taste and dietary habits in the different regions of the British isles (Allen 1968). There are different nutritional risks so different messages are required depending on physiological state—in babies, toddlers, schoolchildren, adolescents, students in bed-sitters, pregnant and lactating women, sedentary middle-aged men, and the housebound elderly.

Since the modern messages have major negative items, anyone embarking on nutrition education is likely to meet lack of interest from politicians, anxiety or delay by civil servants, apathy from the medical profession, a tough counter-attack by the producers and processors of the food(s) you think people should eat less of, and confusion or indifference from the general public. There is a temptation to accept help—money, visual aids, and lobbying—from one of the food producers or processors whose commodity you wish to encourage. To do so carries the grave risk of damaging a nutrition expert's credibility (Ahrens 1977).

Even the proposal to fluoridate drinking water, which has the support of the WHO, our own Department of Health, the Royal College of Physicians, the British Dental Association, etc., etc., continues to meet furious opposition, though no one's job is threatened by it.

To whom then can the nutritional scientist turn for support? Others of the same view, without commercial involvement? But they are enthusiasts (not open-minded); crusaders! Or moderates in the health food movement? No, they are cranks and don't really understand nutritional science.

There is a reorientation in health care, to emphasize healthier personal habits (including diet) in place of medical technology, treating the sick. There has been enthusiasm for community health dietetics/nutrition. But the scepticism and outright opposition to anything which goes beyond 'a balanced diet and prevention of obesity' are formidable. No primer has been drafted comparable to Ritchie's (1967) for developing countries to prepare and guide the innocent nutritionist who emerges from his laboratory with some exciting new results. He wants to help mankind and makes his first appearance on television.

I hope we can pool our experience and develop some honest and fair strategies for tackling this scepticism and opposition in our session.

POSTSCRIPT

I have subsequently suggested (Truswell 1978) that a properly designed nutrition—or other health-education programme—must surely meet three sets of conditions:

first, there must be a consensus of the experts in the country that the message is worth while and needed;

secondly, the advice must be intelligible, practicable (including its economic implications), and safe; and

thirdly, an organization should be set up to monitor and assess its effectiveness.

REFERENCES

Ahlström, A. and Räsänen, L. (1973). Review of food grouping systems in nutrition education. *J. Nutr. Educ.* 5, 13.

Ahrens, R.A. (1977). Out on the 'range', it's credit and credibility that counts. *Nutr. Today* 12, 31.

Allen, D.E. (1968). *British tastes*. Hutchinson, London.

Brock, J.F. and Autret, M. (1952). Kwashiorkor in Africa WHO Monograph Series no. 8. WHO, Geneva.

Burkitt, D.P. (1973). Some diseases characteristic of modern Western civilization. *Br. Med. J.* i, 274.

Hertzler, A.A. and Anderson, H.L. (1974). Food guides in the United States. *J. Am. Diet. Ass.* 64, 19.

Hunt, S.P. (1976). The food habits of Asian immigrants. *Getting the most out of Food* No. 11, pp. 15–51. Van den Berghs & Jurgens, Burgess Hill, West Sussex.

Keys, A. (1952). Human atherosclerosis and the diet. *Circulation* 5, 115.

—— (1968). Official collective recommendations on diet in the Scandinavian countries. *Nutr. Rev.* 26, 259.

Lancet (1977). Editorial: Dietary goals. *Lancet* i, 887.

Ritchie, J.A.S. (1967). *Learning better nutrition. A second study of approaches and techniques.* FAO, Rome.

Staff of the Select Committee on Nutrition and Human Needs, United States Senate (1977). *Dietary goals for the United States,* U.S. Government Printing Office, Washington, D.C. (Stock no. 052-070-039113-2.)

Trowell, H.C. (1972). Ischemic heart disease and dietary fiber. *Am. J. Clin. Nutr.* 25, 926.

Truswell, A.S. (1976). Some micronutrients that may be critical. In *People and food tomorrow*, Hollingsworth, D. and Morse, E. (eds.), p. 57. Applied Science, London.

—— (1977). The need for change in food habits from a medical viewpoint. Paper at Symposium Nutritional Aspects of Food and Agricultural Policies in the U.K. *Proceedings of the Nutrition Society*. (In press.)

—— (1978). A national food policy for prevention of coronary heart disease? *Postgrad. med. J.* 54, 215.

Var föda (1963) Editorial: Mediciniska synpunkter på folkhosten i de nordiska länderna. *Var föda* 20, 3.

Wretlind, A. (1977). General aspects on recommended dietary allowances. Round table on comparison of dietary recommendations in different European countries. 2nd European Nutrition Conference (Munich 15–17 Sept., 1976). *Nutrition & Metabolism* 21, 210.

6 Nutritional problems in changing societies

STANISLAW BERGER

For several reasons the nutrition situation in countries in stages of active development is at present, and no doubt must be in the future, one of the areas of major concern in national as well as global strategy.

The importance and need for appropriate food and nutrition policies, including training, education, extension services, and research in the context of rapidly changing social conditions and economic level, have been recognized in many of these countries, including Poland, since the end of the Second World War.

It is worth noting that an important and stimulatory role in some of these programmes in our country was played by the UNDP/FAO project, 'Research and extension services for food production, processing, and utilization', which was operational in Poland during the period 1963–9.

The declining share of agriculture, both in employment and in producing the national income, transformed these countries from typically agricultural into agro-industrial ones.

The rise in living standards in these countries, and specifically in the rapidly increasing urban population, together with the growth in real wages and incomes result in a constantly higher demand for agricultural products as well as changing food and nutritional patterns. In order to emphasize the nutritional implications of quantity and quality of consumed foods the term, 'food and nutritional patterns', is purposely used in this paper and is preferred to the suggested FAO/WHO (1974) terminology, 'food patterns'. This might be also further justified since, 'nutritional status', refers to the condition of the body resulting from the intake, absorption, and utilization of food and from factors of pathological significance.

The highest demand at present particularly concerns products of animal origin such as meat, milk and fish, as well as refined sugar, compounded fats, white bread and convenience foods. At the same time significant decreases in consumption of cereals and potatoes are observed. Therefore, not only agriculture but also the food processing industry and distribution channels have to cope with these requirements.

It is evident, however that a rise in living standards in economic and technical terms does not automatically improve the nutritional patterns and the nutritional status of the population. I would therefore argue against the prevalent belief of many economists and technocrats that when income is increased considerably nutrition does not require any special attention.

So-called civilization diseases—diseases such as obesity, dental caries, cardiovascular disorders, and so on—are the best examples and evidence supporting this view. I would therefore claim that nutrition-oriented programmes of research and education are needed not only for the hungry and undernourished but also for malnourished well-to-do people.

But in countries where active development is taking place this is of special importance since the food and nutritional patterns—what or how much food or nutrients are consumed per day or per year—depend upon several potentially limiting factors. These include agriculture, food processing capacity, food distribution facilities, and community feeding organizations as well as ingrained food habits. These in turn depend on education, technological progress, and scientific achievements which have been adapted and adjusted specifically to the socio-economic and ecological conditions existing in the countries concerned.

All these factors are strongly and mutually interdependent. Thus our present food and nutritional patterns constitute an integrated feedback system which affects the nutritional status of the population, its development, health, and working efficiency. It is, therefore, often a waste of effort and financial resources when food and nutrition policy is considered separately from the existing and potential food production supply or capacity without careful assessment of nutritional status and food habits among various groups in the population. Control over the whole system is, in my opinion, the key issue to the solution of present and future nutritional problems, particularly in countries where active development is taking place.

INTERRELATIONSHIP BETWEEN AGRICULTURE, FOOD
PROCESSING, STORAGE, AND DISTRIBUTION AND THEIR
NUTRITIONAL IMPLICATIONS

In the past food was normally consumed where it was produced. The more we develop our civilization and have fewer people living on the land the greater are the heavy pressures from modern technology, urbanization, and industrialization. In consequence food supplies take longer to travel from the producer to the consumer. This long journey has, or might have, many significant nutritional implications. They include decrease of nutritive value or contamination during processing, storage, transport, or in the home.

There is no doubt that, generally speaking, food and its nutritional impact in countries where rapid changes in national development are occurring is becoming a very complex issue and needs to be considered in an interdisciplinary and intersectorial way. Therefore, in solving our contemporary and future problems, and in particular improving the quality of consumed food, national food policies based on detailed field surveys must be established in the context of economic and social developments as a pre-condition of any large-scale programme.

It is evident, therefore, that a sound food and nutrition policy must constitute an integral part of a well-planned national policy, having in mind, particularly, long-term implications. It seems desirable that when launching such programmes comprehensive nutritional recommendations for food and nutrition policies should be prepared. Special attention must be given to the agricultural sector. This is particularly relevant at the present time, since in our country as well as in other countries, and especially developing ones, agrarian reforms and agricultural modernization are under way. It would be disastrous if nutritional aspects of such changes were overlooked; and everything possible must be done to ensure that they receive proper consideration. Owing to the importance and impact of agricultural food production and its processing methods on food and nutritional patterns as well as the health of the whole population, the need for nutritional guidelines and highly qualified cadres in agro-industrial programmes is clearly evident.

NEED FOR TRAINING, EDUCATION, AND RESEARCH IN FOOD AND NUTRITION

In those countries where there is a great scarcity of personnel with appropriate nutritional background, particular attention must be given to the training of agriculturalists and other related specialists (veterinarians, agro-allied food technologists, agricultural economists, etc.). They should be aware of, and familiar with, human nutrition and food economics by means of various courses and especially through the inclusion of appropriate curricula within the framework of agricultural colleges and universities.

The introduction of such courses into the training of agriculturalists and other related specialists is of the highest importance in the fight to eradicate hunger and to improve the dietary patterns of the population, as well as in the satisfactory implementation of nutritional guidelines in agriculture and food industries. Although the curricula of colleges and university faculties are often overburdened, many have now been adapted or modified to include the technical advances made in the various sciences that fall within the scope of modern agricultural studies and training. Efforts must also be made to see that as many other educational establishments as possible reshape their courses in the light of this need. Here I would like to emphasize only some general ideas in this connection which might be of some value and worth being discussed.

If one looks at the existing scientific activities and the potential requirements necessary for establishing, guiding, and implementing the previously mentioned programmes the more one realizes how relatively great is the imbalance between the present position and our needs, and how ignorant we really are in this respect.

This is particularly true when one compares other national programmes, e.g. space research, chemistry, energy needs, and electronics, which are receiving not only great financial support but also enjoy the highest priority in national development and implementation.

Therefore in order to accomplish optimal food and nutritional patterns for mankind we badly need to establish, or to develop, existing structures and organizations responsible for training specialists, particularly at the academic level. At the same time we have to stimulate action-oriented research programmes specifically adapted to each country or region where active development is taking place.

In general, however, these programmes should be of an interdisciplinary and flexible character covering all areas of the subjects and at all levels. The *first and second level* should be used as a theoretical background for both basic and applied investigations with particular reference to the role, metabolism, utilization, and interrelationship of various nutrients and other components of foods consumed in the area.

The *third level* should serve for evaluation and determination of optimal nutrient requirements or daily recommended allowances. It should also include food safety and sensory assessment of its relation to body development (both physical and mental), general health, and work efficiency.

The *fourth level* could be of great importance and could play a key role as a main element the management and the establishment of food and nutrition policies at national scale or for specific groups of the population, community feeding systems, education, and extension services. It is evident that for solving our contemporary and also our future nutritional problems, especially in countries where active development is taking place, respective training and research programmes should assume their rightful place in academic and related institutions and receive satisfactory attention.

Specifically, qualified personnel are needed for:

(1) the evaluation of, and advising on, present and future conventional food production as well as for assistance in the formulation of national regional, or world food and nutrition policies;

(2) nutritional evaluation of food marketing and processing methods both at industrial and home levels and new products in relation to consumer protection and health;

(3) teaching food science and nutrition at different levels with particular reference to teacher training institutes, education, and extension services;

(4) managing or co-managing large-scale catering units and other group feeding establishments or central kitchens.

In order to accomplish these objectives respective institutions of training along with research sectors should be established, or developed, at specifically selected academic units, perhaps of an inter-faculty or even inter-university character. As there is not too much experience in this respect I believe it seems desirable that a close co-operation between various universities in different countries should be established and developed. This could be done in many ways including sponsored or assisted programmes by international bodies such as IUNS, IUFoST, or national nutrition societies as well as by the specialized UN agencies.

CONCLUSIONS

Although food and nutrition problems, and particularly optimal nutritional patterns for *Homo sapiens*, should be considered first in terms of what is urgent for the present, it is also important to avoid short-term solutions which may conflict with objectives for the future. Such long-term measures often require much time and adequate resources for real progress and results, but are usually the best in the end. This is particularly true in the case of countries in active development. The experience gained in this field in some countries, including Poland, confirms this approach. I fully agree with the view expressed in a recent editorial in *Nature* that '21st century food needs thought now, and we have only two options available in thinking about future food supplies. The first is to hope that the crunch will not come in our lifetime. The second is to invest heavily in research development and education so that if the crunch does come we can confront it in a prepared and mature way.' This last solution is the only tenable one if we want our civilization to survive and develop towards a better quality of human life throughout the world.

But as is shown in Fig. 6.1 we have approached in a dramatic way a new era in which technological, economic, and social aspects of our life are taking over from ecology, which in the past has influenced our food and nutritional problems. In the figure two phases are

distinguished. Phase I, the past, which lasted around 70 000 generations, and Phase II, the present, comprising only seven generations.

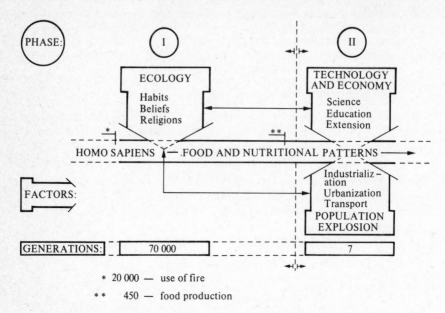

Fig. 6.1. Subordinate factors involved historically in food and nutritional patterns.

It is evident from this approach that, while in the Phase I ecological
and traditional factors played the most important role in creating
the food and nutritional patterns of *Homo sapiens*, our Phase II is
dominated by technology, economic factors, and the explosion of
population together with strong urbanization, industrialization, and
development of transport facilities.

Therefore, in attempting to solve our contemporary and future
nutritional problems these factors should be carefully considered,
analysed, and controlled in order to improve or maintain good food
and nutritional patterns.

The supply of food is at present and no doubt will be in the
future the most important issue for our survival and well-being.
This applies to all of us, but in countries in the stage of active development it should get special attention in order to avoid the pitfalls
and mistakes which took place in our highly industrialized world.

Concerted national and international action is therefore needed
for well-organized programmes aimed at sufficient production,
processing, and utilization of existing and planned food supply in
order to satisfy not only economic but, even more important,

nutritional demands. But in order to formulate and implement food and nutrition policies to this end, intensive research, education and training at all levels, including that for our policy makers, are badly needed.

The sooner we do it the better it will be for all of us and for future generations. We have to face that fact that *Homo sapiens*, who is successfully conquering outer space round our little planet, is still unable to eradicate hunger and malnutrition from our earth.

7 Co-ordination and co-operation in solving nutritional and food problems
HOSSEIN GHASSEMI

It is estimated that close to 500 million people are underfed in the world (UN 1974) and it is apparent that undernutrition and malnutrition are serious problems in the developing regions of Asia, the Far East, the Near East, Africa, and Latin America. Malnutrition is an important cause of mortality among children. There is a high incidence of infectious diseases among young children in most developing countries and the resultant high morbidity and mortality is largely due to lowered body resistance because of malnutrition. Protein energy malnutrition (PEM) is an important cause of child mortality and morbidity and leads to permanent impairment of physical and possibly of mental growth of those who survive. Recent studies have shown that no less than 100 million children under five years of age are affected by moderate to severe PEM (FAO/WHO 1976, p. 9).

On a global basis, other deficiency diseases that deserve high priority action are xerophthalmia, nutrition anaemias, and endemic goitre. In certain geographical areas, notably Africa, rickets continues to be a serious nutrition problem, as are pellagra and zinc deficiency. Inadequate diets that result from extreme inequality in the distribution of food among different socio-economic groups and within families are among major factors responsible.

World-wide appreciation of nutritional problems is a recent phenomenon. Nutrition, in its relatively short history, has made impressive progress. Within a short period of three to four decades a great deal has been learnt about human food consumption and nutritional problems. The methodology of investigation has improved and there is now a much better grasp of the multi-dimensional nature of nutrition problems and much more is known about food, population, urbanization, and health.

Naturally out of all this has grown the urge for problem-solving. During the past twenty years many governments have undertaken nutrition intervention programmes to assist vulnerable groups, aimed particularly at the eradication of protein-energy malnutrition. After two or three decades of experience, there is now doubt as to whether intervention of this type will by itself be effective in controlling nutritional problems. Although there is no systematic analysis at hand to explain the failure, a number of explanations come to mind.

Nutrition has suffered from a low priority status and a wide gap exists between the nutrition worker and the office of the decision-maker. Therefore nutrition programmes have remained a welfare service of very small size with a poor management. Furthermore, overall understanding of the causal relationships in precipitation of nutritional problems has been far from adequate. The causes of malnutrition have been dealt with in a narrow context. Programme formulation has been strikingly non-systematic and nutrition intervention programmes very often lacked clear nutritional objectives. It is interesting to note that, in common practice, a programme often becomes an end rather than a means for achievement of certain objectives.

Even within the philosophy and approach of intervention, there is often a lack of comprehensiveness and entirety in the programmes. For instance, feeding without education, feeding in the absence of infection control, focus on one age group and neglect of others, are among such examples. Nutrition assistance is usually offered in isolation from other social assistance and development efforts. Therefore it provides primarily for symptomatic rather than causal treatment of the problems.

Finally, beneficiaries of nutrition programmes were, in reality, not the vulnerable groups of top priority. A good example is the limited nutrition service provided for infants and pre-school children when access is a major constraint. Very often schoolchildren become the accessible substitute.

Although intervention did not produce the expected impact in terms of control of malnutrition, there certainly were a number of major accomplishments in this brief era. In spite of its shortcomings, nutrition intervention has been instrumental in providing assistance to millions of needy people under most difficult conditions. Furthermore, significant progress was made on various fronts. As mentioned before, worldwide awareness of malnutrition was created, vast amounts of information on food and nutrition accumulated, and analysis of the problem causation improved. Furthermore, numerous institutions for research and training were established and an increasing number of skilled people joined the small core of nutrition workers in developing countries.

Further major progress in this era has been the development of capacity and building of machinery for delivery of nutrition care in both urban and rural areas. On the whole, the expansion and improvement in survey, research, training, service, and promotion which have taken place since the Second World War will undoubtedly serve as a most valuable basis for further progress in the field of nutrition.

CHANGING CONCEPTS

Among major developments in the field of nutrition in recent times two are most significant. The first is the recent appreciation of the multi-factorial nature of nutrition, that is that nutrition is determined by the interaction of a number of factors. Interdisciplinary thinking in the field of nutrition developed as a result of continuous research for a better causal analysis of malnutrition. This has set into motion radical changes in concepts and approaches to the solution of nutrition problems. In the interdisciplinary context, nutrition has experienced a sudden rise in status and there is no doubt that cross-fertilization among various disciplines has been most instrumental in such developments.

As a consequence malnutrition began to be seen as a social problem and not purely as a public-health problem. Nutrition has acquired a great deal of significance as an instrument and outcome of national development. This is a dramatic improvement over the recent past, when nutrition was looked on as only a relief item within the framework of social welfare activities. Therefore, as a parameter in development, nutrition now has to be integrated into the national development planning process. This calls for application of planning techniques to the problems of nutrition. Even more important in this context is the equal emphasis to be given to the treatment of the causes as well as of the symptoms of malnutrition—as a social problem—at the same time. Such an approach represents a drastic departure from the intervention approach in which symptomatic treatment of the problem is focused upon. This brings us to the present era of planning which is the outcome of drastic changes in concepts and approach to the solution of nutritional problems over the last few years.

It is in these recent times that planning for food and nutrition policies and programmes has been strongly advocated. In fact, food and nutrition policies and programmes are a comprehensive and effective multi-disciplinary instrument in integrating nutrition into national development.

At present, matters are in a state of transition. The trend is towards a fully fledged planning situation, where a unified approach for improvement of the food and nutrition situation in developing countries is expected to become effective. Current changes in concepts

and approach naturally open new doors and introduce new difficulties. The prospects are undoubtedly impressive. New trends will
help the status of nutrition to rise further. It is also expected to be
instrumental in closing the gap between the nutrition worker and
the office of the decision-maker. Furthermore, in the new direction
in which we are moving, there will be much more room for systematic thinking and practice. As a result of integration into the
planning process, there will be a sharp focus on objectives, priorities,
selection of alternatives, and strategy of implementation. Food and
nutrition activities are expected to change from a catalogue of
scanty, small and uncoordinated programmes into a single integrated
movement of national proportions. Consequently, increasing support
for nutrition should be generated. This will result in rapid advances
in research, training, organizational development, capacity building,
and leadership.

On the other hand, we know progress means change and change
imposes its own problems. Among the major problems peculiar to
our present transition in the field of nutrition, a few merit special
consideration. The approach to an interdisciplinary subject requires
clear and constructive communication among the disciplines involved.
At the moment, there is a communication problem mainly due to
the absence of a language that could facilitate communication at a
technically satisfactory level within and among the disciplines concerned. Continuous effort from all sides for development of a medium
of satisfactory communication is a fundamental requisite for progress
in an interdisciplinary field. Also, very much related to the communication snags, is a lack of clear understanding of the specific role
of each discipline in the new approach. There will definitely be some
difficulties in arriving at an equilibrium where balanced emphasis is
given to different dimensions of a multidimensional situation such as
nutrition. In other words, the pendulum should hopefully swing to
balance the emphasis with respect to the roles of different disciplines.

The planning and administrative difficulties peculiar to any interdisciplinary
work need hardly be emphasized. Among such difficulties, particular mention
should be made of problems of leadership, organization, simultaneous commitment and financing arrangements among a number of agencies involved. There
is another problem in transition which presents itself with a great deal of complexity. This is the desirable pace of transition in various situations. Our ultimate
purpose is to have fully-fledged and operational food and nutrition policies as
an integrated part and parcel of national development plans (Ghassemi 1976).

CO-ORDINATION

For all practical purposes we are not dealing with a homogeneous situation and the definition of an approach which is both effective in and adaptable to various situations characterized by substantial diversity is a great challenge before us.

As a matter of fact, development of effective machinery for planning and implementation of nutrition activities in a co-ordinated fashion has always been a major concern. A brief review of its evolution would be useful at this point.

In the 1950s establishment of a National Food and Nutrition Council (NFNC) was recommended (FAO/WHO 1962). This council was to be formed of senior officials of the ministries of health, education, agriculture, economy, community development, social welfare, etc. Its tasks included:

(1) Advising the government on food and nutrition problems and the actions to be taken;
(2) Securing agreement on the ways and means through which national programmes can be implemented, whether through the different individual ministries or through the secretariat of the council or through other bodies, e.g. teaching or research centres.

The experience with NFNCs has not been encouraging. In spite of continuous encouragements, NFNCs were either not established or established but not effective (Aylward and Jul 1975). It was later recommended that the NFNC be assisted by a permanent secretariat in a technical and administrative capacity.

A survey in 1973 showed that within 15 years 11 out of 19 countries in the Middle East and North Africa had established NFNCs and only four of them had met more than once a year (Ghassemi 1973).

In the late 1960s, when new concepts emerged and nutrition began to be seen as a parameter in development planning, it was suggested that nutrition like other sectors become a permanent concern of the national planning office and a nutrition unit be established.

Finally, the Ninth WHO/FAO Expert Meeting in 1974 suggested an organizational structure (Fig. 7.1) which encompasses the planning and executive bodies as well as scientific institutions and private industry (FAO/WHO 1976).

Pines (1974), in referring to the political–technical, administrative, and co-ordination barriers involved in formulation and execution of nutrition activities, proposed a review and advocacy approach and calls for short-term improvement of nutrition through systematic review of government policies and programmes by well-placed nutrition advocates, which would ensure necessary adjustments for nutrition purposes.

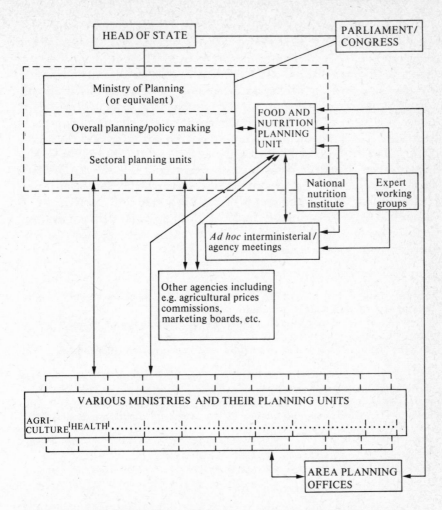

Fig. 7.1. A possible organizational structure for food and nutrition planning. Although the food and nutrition planning unit is shown separately in the diagram it is assumed that in most instances it will be a technical unit within the Ministry of Planning (or its equivalent). As noted in the text, it is desirable that such a unit should relate directly to an official at a level higher than the sectoral divisions of that ministry.

In practice, a fully-fledged operational model such as Fig. 7.1, or even close to that, is non-existent but the trend is quite encouraging. In the recent past, considerable progress has been made in creating awareness of problems and commitment for their solution in various circles and at various levels. The international organizations have been most instrumental and effective in these respect. Also progress made in concepts, methodology, and technology is quite impressive.

At the same time, problems are many. Some are of the opinion that strong commitment at high levels is essential (International Symposium 1977). This may be quite true. There is also no doubt that effective machinery and methodology is an absolute necessity for planning and co-ordination. We know that what was tried did not work as expected and we do not have an effective model in hand. This is to a large extent due to continuous change in approach which itself is a result of continuous search for ways and means of coping with problems of increasing complexity. Co-ordination has always been a matter of serious concern. In 1962 the FAO/WHO Expert Committee on Nutrition emphasized the importance of co-ordination and recommended establishment of NFNCs as a possibly effective instrument. In 1972, during the Dag Hammarskjöld seminar on nutrition, the importance of intimate co-operation in nutrition was emphasized.

REFERENCES

Aylward, F. and Jul, M. (1975). *Protein and nutrition policy in low income countries*. Charles Knight, London.
FAO/WHO Expert Committee on Nutrition (1962). *Sixth report*. Rome.
— (1976). *Ninth report*. Rome.
Ghassemi, H. (1973). *Food and nutrition: regional situation of Second Regional Seminar on Food and Nutrition, Beirut.*
— (1976). *Nutrition policy and program planning in nutrition in the community*. John Wiley, London.
International Symposium on Policies to reduce Nutrition, May 1977.
Pines, J. (1974). Review and advocacy, first steps in nutrition planning. *PAG Document* no. 1. May 1974.
United Nations World Food Conference (1974). *Assessment of the world food situation present and future*. (E. Conf. 65/3) Rome.
Vahlquist, B. (Ed.) (1972). *Nutrition, a priority in African development*. Uppsala.

8 Indigenous foods – their place in human nutrition

FRANCIS AYLWARD

The term 'indigenous' is used in this chapter to describe food supplies from local agronomy, animal production, or wild-life (including fisheries) which are an established part of a local or regional dietary pattern. In this sense the word is used in contrast to imported foods or to new crops or animals which are being introduced.

Many apparently indigenous foods have, of course, been introduced in the past from other countries. One example is the introduction of a variety of crops from Central and South America into Europe and West Africa following the voyages of discovery from Western Europe in the fifteenth and sixteenth centuries. Several West African foods such as cassava, maize, potatoes, and cacao originated in the Americas.

Current discussions on food supplies, especially in the developing world, often stress the importance of the transport of food from one region of the world to another (e.g. from the USA to Africa), the introduction of new crops, or the development of new types of food. While all these have uses and advantages it must be remembered that they have also disadvantages.

It is true that for emergency relief, following natural disasters or man-made emergencies, food supplies in quantity may need to be transported from one region of the world to another. But such transfers, on a long-term basis, may tie the economy of one country to another to an undesirable extent. For this reason most industrialized countries, with some significant exceptions such as the UK and Japan, attempt to obtain their staple foods from local agriculture.

New crops can also play a part in the economy of some countries as can also the development of new varieties of existing crops. But often these new or improved crops take much time to develop and may benefit mainly the more prosperous section of the agricultural community since they will probably benefit primarily those who have, or can supply, the new skills or extra capital which they need for their introduction. Furthermore, such new foods, while being nutritionally advantageous, may not be readily acceptable into an existing dietary pattern.

Expatriate advisers in developing countries have in the past sometimes stressed the need for new crops and new foods as the main
route to nutritional improvement in local diets. In consequence
there has been a considerable investment in many countries in
respect of such projects both in terms of capital and human resources by local governments and also by international bodies.

Projects like these have only a limited interest in research and
development studies of existing foods. In part this may be because
there is more scientific 'glamour' in the work on new foods and
in part because work on local foods may not so readily receive
financial support from national and international bodies. In the
same way local foods may receive inadequate attention in nutrition
education programmes. Indeed sometimes there is more emphasis
given to the disadvantages of such foods, e.g. cassava, than to the
advantages, e.g. low cost, adaptability, and dietary acceptance.

ASPECTS OF STUDIES ON LOCAL FOODS

In spite of what has just been said it would be incorrect to give the
impression that no work at all has been done on the wide range of
local foods available in the different regions of the world. It has to
be remembered that these foods form the staple foods of almost all
the people in many countries and that many millions of people
rarely consume 'western-type' foods.

Studies which have been done include analysis, effect of food
preparation and cooking on vitamin and mineral content, and dehydration methods. For example a very extensive survey of the foods
of Mexico and central American countries by Harris and his colleagues
at MIT in the 1940s showed the value of these foods in respect of
vitamin and mineral contents. Similar work has been done in Nigeria
and other countries of West Africa and studies on the use of vegetables
in Uganda have been made by various workers.

Several authors have drawn attention to the use of (to the Western
mind) unusual sources of animal foods such as insects and large bats
while studies have been carried out in West Africa on the large
rodents, e.g. cane-rats, and also on the giant snail.

As with all other foods the nutritional value when it is consumed
will be different from that in its fresh state and its value may be
enhanced or diminished by pre-cooking preparation or by processing
in the factory or kitchen. Harris drew attention to the fact that in
Mexico the traditional method of preparing the tortilla began with
the soaking of the maize in lime-water followed by wet milling. It

was shown that the liberation of *bound* nicotinic acid in this process could be one reason why pellagra was rare in Mexico in contrast to other maize-eating regions. In addition the lime-water treatment increased the calcium content of the maize products. Aylward noted that in Ghana maize was wet-milled following a soaking (fermentation) process.

The value of preparation techniques has been recognized in other foods for many years including the elimination of cyanides from cassava, destruction of enzyme-inhibitors in legumes, and reduction of factors related to favism in broad beans.

Work on fermented-food preparations has also been carried out by van Veen in the Netherlands and by Platt in the United Kingdom. It has also been done extensively on soy products by various workers in Eastern Asia.

More recently, too, increased attention has been given to fermented animal products such as soft cheeses and yoghurts and similar lactic fermentations. Rather surprisingly very little work so far appears to have been done on the many alcoholic fermented beverages which can make a useful contribution to nutritional status in terms of vitamin intake.

FOOD HABITS AND PREFERENCES

This is still a neglected field although it has more recently attracted some attention. A recent (UK/Nigeria) paper gave some details of a study of meat preferences in Nigeria and showed differences from the traditional pattern of acceptance in Europe in that there were marked preferences for tough (chewable) meat rather than for the tender ('soft') cuts. An earlier study in Ghana by Jollens had given similar results.

It is clear that there is a need for more surveys like this if adequate and worthwhile programmes are to be established to obtain nutrionally improved dietary habits.

APPLICATION TO NUTRITION EDUCATION PROGRAMMES

In the light of the information given in this paper it is clear that those concerned with nutrition education should prepare for themselves adequate bibliographies of work already carried out in their own country. At the same time there is scope for new projects at different educational levels. Some projects will require access to equipment for analysis for samples of foodstuffs; other projects require virtually no specialized equipment but depend on the systematic collection of information on dietary habits and food intake levels.

Section II
The educational background

9 Food and nutrition education and training: an introduction to the theme

FRANCIS AYLWARD

INTRODUCTION

We are concerned in this chapter with two main themes:

(1) the content of food and nutrition education; and
(2) the educational competencies and the administrative structures available to promote them.

All the papers on the content of nutrition education apply equally to both the formal and non-formal sectors, and the papers on educational methods and techniques will also apply across the educational scene.

The question of what should be taught in nutrition, as well as the question of programme planning, evaluation, and co-ordination, applies to all categories and levels of education.

The above-mentioned themes may furthermore be considered in terms of industrialized countries and also in relation to the developing world, with the recognition that there is no clear line of demarcation. Many countries or areas within countries are in transitional stages of development; moreover, within the so-called industrialized countries (for example in Europe), there may be many regions of 'underdevelopment'.

This chapter is designed as an introduction to the more specialized papers dealing with relevance in education, educational methods, administrative problems, and co-operation, but three general comments may be made about the content of nutrition education on the whole:

(1) with the advances of knowledge over the past few decades, we must avoid dogmatism in nutrition teaching; there are now many areas of keen debate on the application of nutritional science to practical dietary problems.
(2) there is also a much greater recognition of the importance of linking nutrition, considered as a laboratory or clinical science, with the human and social sciences; and
(3) arising from (1) and (2) it will be accepted that many of the simplified ideas in older textbooks and information on this subject must be modified with changes in emphasis, more especially when used in countries with different cultural patterns.

TERMINOLOGY : FOOD AND NUTRITION STUDIES

The term 'nutrition', and its equivalent in different languages, is used in different senses by different authors. In the broad sense, it may be used to cover the study of:

(1) foods, including food composition and changes in composition from source to consumer;
(2) biochemical and physiological processes taking place within the body in health and disease; and
(3) social and economic questions relating to food sources and supplies and to food habits.

There is an even broader area which includes the nutrition of animals—particularly farm animals—and plant nutrition.

Often (and especially in languages other than English) the term nutrition, or human nutrition, is used primarily in sense (2) with a stress on physiological aspects; in this sense it may be interpreted in a medical and public-health context. No one would deny the central importance of health aspects of nutrition, and related work on practical dietetics, but a restriction to public health questions may discourage ministries and organizations outside the health field from taking an interest in nutrition. As a consequence, national nutrition programmes, involving food, agriculture, and also education, may be retarded, with the result that nutritional measures in preventive medicine may lack the necessary backing.

In order to avoid these difficulties and to emphasize the broader aspects of human nutrition, an increasing number of authors in English are using a combined term, e.g. food and nutrition science, or food science and nutrition. French authors appear to be using composite terms, such as 'alimentation-nutrition'. This question of terminology is important and needs to be clarified by further discussion.

A further difficulty of terminology in different languages and in different parts of the UN system occurs in the use of the word, 'education'. The term nutrition education is sometimes limited to activities in the adult education area and the word, 'training' to organized courses (often of brief duration). Many university-level courses, e.g. in science, medicine, and agrigulture, provide, however, both a broad general 'education' and also 'training' in preparation for a profession.

In a report prepared for Unesco (Aylward 1972), the title, 'Food and Nutrition Education and Training' was used to ensure that the twin aspects of professional and other courses could be emphasized. In this book the term nutrition education can be regarded as a convenient summary of a longer title.

FORMAL AND NON-FORMAL EDUCATION

We can distinguish between two areas of education, one within the formal system (see Table 9.1) of primary, secondary, and tertiary institutions, the other embracing adult education or extension activities (see Table 9.2).

There is no simple word in English to describe this second sector, which is concerned with the dissemination of knowledge among the general public, irrespective of age group. The term 'non-formal' may be used as convenient shorthand for a wide range of educational exchange including adult education, community development, extension services, and so on.

TABLE 9.1

Sectors of the educational system

Institutions concerned or potentially concerned with
food and nutrition studies

Pre-primary and
primary schools

Secondary ⎱   General
schools ⎰   Vocational

Tertiary

The university sector including centres of university rank under various names		*The non-university sector* including a wide variety of institutions
1 Faculties, colleges, or schools of:	**2** College of education (Teacher training colleges) which may be inside or outside the university system. Colleges may include:	**3** 'Mono-technics', or federal or general institutions concerned with subjects such as:
(a) Liberal arts	(a) Independent general colleges	(a) Dietetics, nursing, public health
(b) Science, including science-based departments of nutrition and/or food science	(b) Independent specialized centres (e.g. for home economics)	(b) Agriculture, veterinary studies and fisheries
(c) Dietetics	(c) University departments or school	(c) Food industries: food processing and food technology
(d) Medicine and public health		(d) Home economics
(e) Home economics		(e) Catering, institutional or hotel management
(f) Agriculture and veterinary science		

TABLE 9.2

*The diffusion of information outside the formal educational
system—non-formal and extension*

(a) Areas

Health and para-medical programmes including physical education	Agriculture, community development, and related programmes	General education programmes	Other areas

Note: Nutrition is often a component of wider health or other programmes.

(b) Agencies

Ministries, e.g. Education, Health and Social Welfare, Food and Agriculture, Community Development.	Local government	Voluntary or professional bodies	Educational institutions	Organizations concerned with media

(c) Communications media

Classroom or other groups	Printed word Books and pamphlets Newspapers and magazines Advertisements	Radio Cinema Television Visual aids	Project techniques

It is probably unwise to make too sharp a distinction between the sectors—interchanges of experience and techniques can be of the greatest value. Some of the techniques (for example the use of films and more recently of television) were stimulated in several countries in relation to non-formal education, but now have an established place within the classroom.

On the other hand there are administrative and other differences between to two sectors. Formal education is usually well-established within the framework of a national Ministry of Education, or its equivalent; non-formal education may be promoted by a variety of bodies and (in respect of food and nutrition) ministries such as health and agriculture; professional and industrial bodies may make important contributions.

THE IMPORTANCE OF THE FORMAL EDUCATION SYSTEM

The reason why there is a particular concern about nutrition in formal education may be summarized as follows:

1. In all countries, even the less developed ones, there is in existence a formal educational system and usually a Ministry of Education and local education authorities. Efforts have been made in a number of countries, and perhaps especially in developing countries, to establish new types of organization. There is, however, everything to be said, on grounds of prudence and economy, for using to the full the educational system as it exists and for making such modifications as may be necessary.

2. Nutrition is regarded in some countries as relevant only to Ministries of Health and Agriculture. In developing countries (and in some industrialized countries) there may be no person qualified in nutrition in any senior position in the Ministry of Education or in key educational centres, such as colleges of education for the training of teachers. It is important, therefore, that Ministries of Education should recognize the importance of nutrition and the potentialities of the educational system in contributing to improvements in health through the teaching of nutrition.

3. At the present time there is rethinking in many countries on the content of science education and there is room for the introduction of ideas regarding food and nutrition in new curricula. Rethinking is taking place also in other areas such as health education, physical education, environmental and ecological studies, and home economics; this is an appropriate time to examine the possibility of linking food and nutrition studies with other subjects.

4. Over and above these points is the question of training professional nutritionists in the universities, and training teachers familiar with nutritional ideas in colleges of education at both university and sub-university levels. This point is examined in a little more detail later; there is good evidence that many of the difficulties in promoting nutritional programmes in developing countries arise from the shortage of qualified trained personnel.

The remainder of this introduction is devoted to a brief examination of the place of nutrition in different sectors within the formal educational system.

FOOD AND NUTRITION STUDIES IN THE PRE-PRIMARY, PRIMARY, AND SECONDARY SCHOOL SYSTEMS

The reasons for the introduction of food and nutrition studies in the curricula of schools may be justified as follows:

(1) to make a contribution to general education;
(2) to assist in the promotion of better food habits and nutritional standards within families and local communities;
(3) to assist on a long-term basis in promoting a sound public opinion on food and nutrition questions; and
(4) to encourage some proportion of the school population to take up professional, or para-professional, careers (including teaching) related directly or indirectly to food and nutrition.

The following questions are important:

(a) at what stage, in terms of age groups, should food and nutrition teaching be introduced?
(b) what should be the lines of approach in relation to other subjects, such as:
    natural sciences—particularly chemistry and biology;
    health education and physical education;
    agricultural and rural studies;
    history, geography, and social studies;
    home economics;
(c) what are the special problems in relation to vocational education?
(d) what should be the curricula in relation to (b) and (c)?

COLLEGES OF EDUCATION : CENTRES FOR THE TRAINING OF TEACHERS

Types of institution

There are many different types of institution, including those concerned with teacher training at sub-university level, those which have integrated degree courses, and those which provide education courses for graduates in different subjects as a preparation for a career in teaching. Further distinctions can be made between colleges offering courses of a general nature and those working in a more limited field, e.g. home economics, agriculture. Other distinctions can be made, depending on whether the college functions on a university campus as a department of a university or is independent of the university sector. The administrative patterns, and also the patterns of courses and curricula, in industrialized countries vary from one country to another; similar wide variations occur in developing countries. There may also be considerable differences within institutions in any one country.

Potential importance of colleges of education in relation to nutrition and food studies

Proposals to introduce food and nutrition teaching in schools are likely to be ineffective in any one country unless there is sustained support from appropriate colleges of education (or university departments of education), as well as from local and national administrators. The colleges or equivalent university departments can be key centres for changes in educational curricula. They can make a contribution to food and nutrition studies in various ways. First, through their regular courses for students preparing for careers in teaching. Secondly, through the provision of vacation or special courses and seminars for serving teachers. Thirdly, in acting as centres for information and advice; and fourthly, in sponsoring adult education activities.

Among the questions which should be discussed and to which answers need to be found relate to:

(1) the place of food and nutrition studies in different types of course;
(2) curricula for students who have first degrees in nutrition, food science, home economics, or related subjects;
(3) the relation of food and nutrition studies to other subject (see Table 9.3); and
(4) links between teaching programmes and the related activities noted in Table 9.3, namely school health services, school meal programmes, and school garden/food-production projects.

Food and nutrition programmes in industrialized countries have often been science-based; there is now increasing interest in links with the social sciences (see Table 9.4). These links are of potential importance in colleges of education in both industrialized and developing countries.

UNIVERSITIES AND OTHER INSTITUTIONS OF UNIVERSITY STATUS: OTHER INSTITUTIONS IN THE TERTIARY SECTOR OF EDUCATION

Importance in relation to food and nutrition studies

In the context of this Conference, the tertiary sector of education is important as a source of specialists for lectureships in colleges of education and for teaching posts in schools. But the activities of universities and other tertiary institutions have, of course, wider implications which include:

(1) the training of specialists for a variety of posts—administrative, managerial, research, extension, and advisory—within the local or national government service, or within the private sector of food and associated industries;
(2) the wider education of students of medicine and public health, of agriculture and veterinary science, of food science, food technology, home economics, and other subjects who should have some knowledge of human nutrition to be applied in their professional work; and
(3) the wider education of other graduates (e.g. in economics and the social sciences) who, in adminstrative and other positions, may be responsible for the formulation or execution of policies or for the formation of public opinion.

Apart from questions of the planning of courses and the development of curricula, there are many points which require detailed consideration, including:

(1) the place of departments of human nutrition (and/or food science and/or food and nutrition science) within universities and parallel institutions in industrialized and in developing countries;
(2) the place of nutrition in medical and public health curricula and in the courses designed for professions ancillary to medicine (for example, dieticians for hospitals and for public health activities);

TABLE 9.3

Food and nutrition studies in colleges of education

Sections	Some objectives
(a) *Food and nutrition topics*	
(1) Natural sciences	To supply as required a *scientific* background at appropriate levels in chemical and microbiological aspects of foods, and in biochemical and physiological aspects of nutrition.
(2) Social sciences including history, geography, and social anthropology	To supply the social science background to food and nutrition studies with illustrations from the life of the individual, the family, and the local and national communities.
(3) Family and health aspects (including physical education)	To relate (i) and (ii) to local problems and to provide surveys of the effects of undernutrition and malnutrition or both in local communities.
(4) Food production and utilization: local agriculture, fisheries, and wildlife as sources of foods: food consumption patterns	To provide a detailed picture of the local, regional, and national situation within a given country, including surveys of local foods and food habits.
(5) International aspects	To consider food and nutrition problems in their world setting and to outline the activities of the United Nations agencies and of international scientific and other technical co-operation and professional bodies.
(b) *Educational competencies*	
(1) General	To provide knowledge and understanding of pedagogical principles underlying aspects of educational development.
(2) Special	To provide competencies specifically related to the teaching of nutrition with particular reference to educational methods and materials.
(c) *Related activities*	
(1) School meals	
(2) School gardens	To provide practical experiences in support of classroom learning activities.
(3) School health services	

TABLE 9.4

*Food and nutrition science in relation to social and
economic studies*

University or other departments or research centres	Example of activities
History (including the history of science, technology, and agriculture)	Food production and utilization at different stages in history. History of food habits. Interaction of food supplies and other events; explorations, opening up of new regions; famines.
Geography	Food production and food patterns in different localities, countries, and regions. Effects of local environmental conditions (including climate and soils).
Social anthropology	Food habits, including taboos and their relation to local cultures.
Psychology	Food preferences and food acceptibility. Factors leading to changes in habits.
Economics	Relation of food supplies to general economic conditions. Relation between food, health, and income levels for individuals, families, and communities. Problems of rural and urban development and migration from country to town. Food marketing. Patterns of internal and international trade.
Statistics	Application of statistical methods to agricultural production and to food distribution and consumption.
Epidemiology	Comparative studies of health and disease in different localities and correlation with food supplies and food patterns.
Educational studies	Place of food and nutrition in the general, professional, and adult education system. Relationship of nutrition to learning ability.

(3) the place of human nutrition in other courses, such as agriculture and home economics;

(4) the relation of nutrition teaching to research programmes; and

(5) methods for increasing the supply of specialists in food and nutrition for teaching at different levels.

The tertiary sector of education includes not only universities and institutions of university rank, but a variety of institutions operating at the sub-professional level; in many countries these institutions are important in the training of paramedical personnel, and also of personnel for agriculture, the food industries, and the catering and hotel industries. In respect of food and nutrition, questions arise similar to those listed above.

GENERAL OBSERVATIONS

The purpose of this introduction is to indicate topics which are important in relation to the general theme of this section. In many countries—especially developing countries—there is a shortage of people with adequate training in nutrition for teaching both within the formal educational system and in non-formal education, as well as for other posts in public health, in the food industries and elsewhere. It is hoped that in our discussions some attention can be given to priorities in action and to methods of co-operation between individuals and institutions in the industrialized and in the developing world. This co-operation, if it is to be successful, will involve not only the interchange of information and the transfer of techniques from one country to another, but a recognition that methods must be modified and adapted to meet new and local situations. This point is true for several branches of knowledge; it is particularly important when we are considering nutrition in local and national cultures.

REFERENCES

Aylward, F. (1972). *Food and nutrition education and training—with particular reference to general education systems in developing countries.* UNESCO ED/WS/353 October 1972.

10 The need-identification process: the question of educational relevance

ISAIAS RAW

In the last decade educational planning and implementation have evolved a more rational approach based on the system analysis of problems, goals, resources and priorities that define behavioural objectives around which the curriculum and evaluations are designed. Utilizing this approach in the introduction or innovation of nutrition education, one must precede this process with the identification of the nutritional problems to be addressed. From this one would derive the objectives which can be achieved through education. These objectives must then be translated into the development of a proper curriculum, adequate not only for the problems to be faced, but for the cultural and socio-economic characteristics of the target population as well. This is more easily stated than executed. It is no wonder that nutrition education has run into many failures and a great deal of criticism. Let us attempt to analyse some of the steps in this process, and identify problems and pitfalls.

IDENTIFICATION OF PROBLEMS

The first step is the actual identification of the nutritional problems that form the base for selection of priorities in nutrition education. In most cases these problems are part of the total social complex, involving the socio-political and economic structure, education and technological level, religious and traditional beliefs, population density and growth, and ecological factors. As shown in Fig. 10.1, it is not possible, and frequently not even necessary, to isolate causes and consequences, but one must select intervention points that are feasible and that will contribute to the promotion of the desired changes.

The educator must rely on the results of surveys and research. One needs not only valid data, but proper analysis that can only be carried out by a multidisciplinary team which includes public-health specialists, agricultural experts, economists, planners, and politicians. The interaction of experts of diverse backgrounds allows for a combined view from different perspectives, thus providing a greater chance of obtaining a more objective analysis of the problems of the proposed interventions, their priorities, implications, and chances of success.

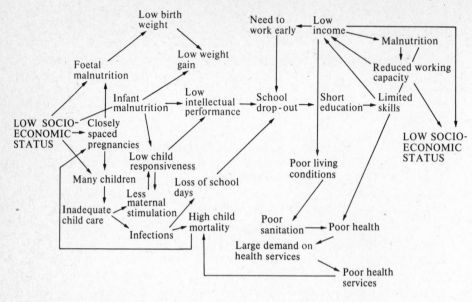

Fig. 10.1. Factors contributing to the low level of education of the nutritionally deprived population.

Even this collective analysis cannot guarantee a correct interpretation, specifically in instances where basic scientific information is not established. An example of this was the 1955 UN decision, based on an inflated idea of the minimum nitrogen requirements of the body, to place world-wide priority on the increase of the production and intake of proteins.

Particularly important for the educator are the findings which have proved that there is an intellectual deficit in those who have suffered severe malnutrition during foetal life and early infancy. Although these findings substantiate the impact of early malnutrition on intellectual development, we have no clear data on its irreversibility —data which would set special educational goals for the population exposed to these conditions. Figure 10.1 shows that there are many other factors contributing to the low level of education of the nutritionally deprived population.

In contrast to other disciplines where the goals are generally valid throughout a country, nutrition education is mission-oriented and must provide specific education to help solve specific problems. In most cases a national overview does not provide a detailed picture of the nutrition problems, nor the specific goals of nutrition education. This is evident not only when we compare rural and metropolitan areas, but even within the newly developed metropolitan areas themselves. As a transitory result of the developmental process, they are inhabited by a range of populations with different problems. While one extreme suffers from one form of malnutrition—obesity, cardiovascular disease and its consequences—the other extreme group corresponds to the undernourished or children of poor working parents, who are affected in increasing numbers by marasmus that will leave them physically and mentally handicapped.

GOALS AND TARGETS

Analysis of the nutritional problems will not only identify the specific problems of the different socio-economic groups, but will also indicate within each group the age and sex sub-groups that are most susceptible. It might be infants who are more affected by the protein-caloric deprivation, adolescents who develop atherosclerosis lesions, or women who develop iron-deficient anaemia. This analysis will also establish priorities by selecting the sub-groups that are more affected and those, such as children, in whom the consequences are most profound and lasting.

USE OF EDUCATION

Once the nutritional goals and the target groups are defined, the next problem is actually to decide if these goals are best achieved, or achieved at all, within the constraints of time and resources, by education.

There are, for example, a number of goals that are more rapidly and efficiently achieved by other methods. Iron, iodine, vitamins, and other micronutritients can be added to staple foods, spices, or water, and in that way no active effort or conviction is required of anyone in order to consume the recommended amounts.

Education is a structured process that aims at providing rational understanding and that creates a new way of analysing facts and information. It is this acquisition of a capacity for analysis, synthesis, and generalization that may result in a conscious change in behaviour.

FOOD HABITS

This brings us to food patterns and practices, which as everyone knows are extremely resistant to change. Social anthropologists claim that this is particularly true for staple foods. It is certainly slow, but changes have occurred in the last two centuries: wheat from the Fertile Crescent is the main staple food in North America, potato and corn from America the staple food in parts of Europe, and Asian rice the staple food in Latin America.

Today these changes must occur at a very fast rate if one expects to meet nutritional requirements under given conditions and adjust them to changing food situations. Thus, changing nutrition habits is a main expectation of and challenge to nutrition education—but there is no substantial evidence that this goal has ever been achieved.

At higher levels, nutrition education is part of the scientific background and should appeal to objectivity and rationality. It can and should challenge some traditional preconceptions.

In general education it is much harder to present the full scientific evidence and it is advisable to avoid the simple polemics of challenging religious beliefs and traditional habits if they are not essential to the achievement of the proposed goals. It is important for the educator to realize that some of the traditions inherited from almost pre-historic times may represent a process of perpetuating essential information to a non-scholarly, non-scientific society, and that this information is correct and useful under some conditions. Not only was primitive man able to develop domesticated plants and animals—an achievement on a scale rarely repeated since then—but through tradition preserved important discoveries, such as planting and eating beans with maize, or treating the maize with calcium hydroxide to improve its nutritional value. Avoiding milk for adults represents a learned behaviour for populations with high incidence of lactase deficiency. The Indian peasant who does not eat the cow has created a closed cycle with efficient use of solar energy, while advanced Western farming cannot exist without the input of fossil fuel. To be aware of and sensitive to local culture and recognize the adequate intervention it is essential to develop and use local talent.

LIMITATIONS OF EDUCATION

One must be candid in admitting the limitations of all educational processes. We can transmit knowledge and students will acquire a sophisticated reasoning process and a large baggage of information that they assimilate and accept as true. Still, education often does not achieve its final goal: the transfer of reasoning capability and critical evaluation of information in daily, non-professional life. Unfortunately it is exactly this that nutrition education seeks.

What we frequently see is the coexistence within a single individual of two cultures: one acquired through education and the other the 'traditional' culture, the latter frequently determining the actual daily behaviour of individuals, including their food habits. This 'traditional' culture is not exclusively one of long-standing beliefs transmitted from previous generations, but also the 'hearsay' culture generated in all societies that frequently acquires more power than formal education. It is this which explains why some of our students consume 'natural food', high amounts of vitamins or 'protein supplements', which signifies a rapid change in food habits among the most educated young population in the world, and which has a profound nutritional impact.

Thus the challenge for nutrition education is not simply to change nutrition habits formed generations ago, but also to prevent the acquisition of other irrational attitudes towards nutrition which result from new, pseudo-scientific information.

NUTRITION ADVICE

The above definition of education is very restrictive and includes the ideal and most sophisticated type of learning. Although this is the goal for all levels, in the lower levels education is mostly an authoritarian transmittal of information. Authoritarian education does not provide the critical capacity to deal with changing situations, but it does have an important pragmatical role, not just in the lower levels of schooling (frequently all the education that the majority of the population at risk will ever receive), but for adults as well.

Nutrition advice and information must not and should not be restricted to formal education. It should take advantages of the mass-communication media and learn from the techniques developed for consumerism, which, for instance, have been successful in persuading, in a very short time, most of the world's population to spend part of their food budget on cola-flavoured drinks.

A very simple form of nutrition education is the actual demonstration of the preparation of food and tasting of the finished product. This technique is often used by industry in the introduction of new products, and can be used to promote the introduction of balanced meals or the utilization of newly introduced crops (either new and different strains, or even different species). Used to promote 'commerciogenic' products, it can be re-directed to improve dietary intakes without further assaulting the budget limitations that in most cases are the ultimate cause of nutrition deficiency.

TYPES OF INTERVENTION

An effective approach is to convey nutrition education through a number of channels, including formal and non-formal education, as a co-ordinated programme. Preceding this implementation of nutrition education programmes other educational goals are essential: the re-training of teachers for all educational levels and categories including technical education, medical, public health, and para-medical professionals, and agricultural personnel, who will act as channels to convey nutrition advice to the population at risk.

Especially important is the proper education for the future and persuasion of the present political and economic leadership. This is critical in several developing countries where nutrition interventions are being postponed while priority is given to economic development that, at best, would trickle down to improve mass nutrition. Anyone with a proper background in nutrition knows that a very small investment in food supplementation could erase the permanent blindness which is due to vitamin-A deficiency, or cure and prevent the marked decrease of physical capability that results from iron deficiency. These are some of the common nutrition problems in developing countries which cripple the economic development at the expense of the well-being and life of millions.

Thus, nutrition education has a relevant role in any nutrition intervention and must be a co-ordinated and connected action which will reach the ruling classes and their future replacements, the health-nutrition professionals (medical doctors, nurses, dieticians), food production specialists (agronomists and food technologists), teachers, students, and the general public. Although the ultimate goals of different education interventions may be the same, the specific goals are different and must be adequate with regard to the level of sophistication and content for each sub-set of goals.

Such a concerted action, where nutrition education is a complement, is always a large project, demanding large sums of money and a large cadre of specialists. International institutions and funding agencies are geared for this large-scale, complex operation and carefully scrutinize the proposed project through a no less elaborate, complex, and costly pre-investment feasibility study. Although this is one pathway to attack the problem, it is not the only pathway, nor is it the most successful. The more needy countries may not be able to establish large programmes owing to cost and manpower limitations. There is certainly room for a very large number of limited nutrition interventions which, properly devised and conducted, may have a large impact. It is the expertise of the leaders of these more limited but successful interventions that is necessary for the larger projects.

Once the nutrition interventions which will attempt to address the existing nutrition problems are selected, the next step is the preparation of their actual content, be it a curriculum or a message. Although this seems to be the domain of the teacher or the mass communication media expert, it requires a variety of expertise and experts, the range of which may cover not just the basic scientific rationale, but economics, sociology, food production, agronomy, etc.

Again, this is the product of a collective effort which would look very deeply into the proposed interventions and their implications.

FORMAL NUTRITION EDUCATION

Nutrition education should be introduced at all levels of formal education. It will make its greatest impact in the formative years, when children are curious and youngsters are concerned about themselves. In my experience, the best method of motivation is to centre these programmes on discussion and analysis of the students' own nutritional problems and dietary habits.

There is no room in the present curriculum for the addition of a separate discipline of nutrition. The natural thing to do, however, is to combine it with science education, which becomes relevant, personalized, and exciting; food and nutrition being a good theme which provides for the sound learning of scientific attitude and principles. This should be a challenge for the co-operation of centres for science education development which evolved in the 1960s and have experienced available local talents.

Frequently the teaching of nutrition at the university level is restricted to dieticians and nurses. Although these professionals apply their acquired knowledge, they almost invariably do not transmit it, thus reaching for a limited time (such as in lunch programmes or during hospitalization) a small segment of the population. In contrast, it is an almost universal fact that medical students, who must learn to recognize the social realities within which they will practise and must be prepared to help their patients recover and maintain health, do not have any formal course in nutrition. The introduction of nutrition in the medical curricula is a priority for developed and developing countries, as is the preparation of paramedical professionals who, with the physician, would be efficient conveyers of nutrition education and advice.

RELEVANCE

The two main points to remember in the development of materials for nutrition education are that the material itself should be relevant to the daily lives of the people using it and that the vehicle used for transmitting this material should be suited to the intended audience. That is, the material must not just provide basic principles, but information that can be translated into action as well. It should take into account the economic system, the purchasing power of the target population, the availability of different foods, the level of food technology, the social structure, food practices, and religious beliefs. The vehicle used should be adequate for the message and for the target population. Written information cannot reach illiterates; television messages will not reach the semi-starving, nor convince them to improve their diets.

No nutrition education programme can be transferred from one nation to another and in all cases it should be tailored to the specific environment (large city, peripheral slum, village, or rural area).

CONCLUSIONS

Nutrition and food patterns and practices are deep-rooted in the general living conditions and culture of a country. Basic knowledge about the nature of vitamins, proteins, and other nutrients can be cross-culturally transferred, but the application of this knowledge to local conditions must be determined on the spot.

In this chapter an attempt has been made to deal with the process of identification of nutrition and food problems and needs related to the individual, community, and the country in general and how these problems can best be solved in the context of locally available resources. This analysis reflects two major aspects: (a) the human nutritional need problems and the fulfilment of these, and (b) the nutrition and food situation in the community and country and factors affecting this situation. In drawing upon the knowledge and experience of various categories of professional resource people and documentation (surveys, research, etc.), the nutrition problem/concept is formulated. The involvement of politicians, parents, children and lay people in general should be sought. The impact of the levels of educational technology and available educational facilities on programme development is dealt with in other chapters of this book.

11 Curriculum design for nutrition education

GARY A. GRIFFIN

INTRODUCTION

This chapter will consider curriculum planning for nutrition education programmes in schools. Although I am aware that there are other agencies of society which educate—television, radio, the church, social and civic organizations, museums, and the like—it is through the formal institution of the school that most of the people of the world come into contact with specific instruction which is tied to specific outcomes (Cremin 1977). Schools, whether for very young children or for adults, are societal institutions charged with bringing about a knowing, caring, skilful populace. It should be noted, however, that the curriculum planning modes that I will be discussing can be adopted by other formal agencies or employed in less formal educational settings.

CURRICULUM PLANNING AS CONTROL

At the outset I believe it is important to acknowledge that curriculum planning is an exercise in the control of people, events, places, time, energy, knowledge, skill, and other related phenomena. That is, when one plans that students will have certain educational contacts—in this instance, the content and skill related to nutrition science—one, by definition, has chosen *not* to attend to other phenomena. Put another way, given the limited time and energy resources available to teachers and students, planning for the interaction of those teachers and students controls their behaviour. As we suggest certain outcomes of nutrition education programs we are at the same time implicitly suggesting that other, unplanned-for outcomes are not as important as the ones we include in our curriculum. As we suggest that students do certain things, read certain printed materials, write and report about certain phenomena or produce certain products, we are controlling the students' time and energy and eliminating from their present lives other opportunities to read, to do, to write and report about, and so forth (Tyler 1950).

When one considers that a curriculum plan is a major form of social control, the importance of a sound, reliable, and widely accepted system of values becomes critical. Certainly, when one believes that the social, cultural, political, and economic ramifications of a people's knowledge and skill as such apply to the concepts undergirding reasoned and sensitive use of the environment—specifically that which is consumable, for purposes of this conference—one must make critical control decisions. What values will inform what we plan for and with young persons and adults? What evidence can we garner which will support the use of these values as criteria for selection of one piece of knowledge or skill into or out of our curriculum? How can we continue to justify the curriculum we present as it is tested over time?

The curriculum issue here is that we must be able to justify, to rationalize, and to monitor our curricular decisions—whatever they may be—according to a strongly and clearly stated value position. This is not nearly as easy as it sounds. First, it is not easy because it is not a behaviour that we are accustomed to using. We most often present a curriculum or an instructional programme as though it had sprung fully grown from the forehead of Zeus. A curriculum is too often the listing of certain activities for students and teachers with little or no systematic attention given to why such activities are presented.

Secondly, the value positions which may appear to support the inclusion or exclusion of certain curriculum elements are open to social, political, and economic question. Especially in countries which are characterized by a multi-cultural, multi-ethnic populace, we find that one person's values are another person's poisons, to mix a metaphor. The argument here centres around the concept of clarification of values. How much do those who plan curricula know about the persons who will use them? Is there a system of values that both groups share? Are there conflicts in values between the planning persons and the users? If there are conflicts, how can they be resolved? How powerful are the conflicts in terms of the potential utility of the curriculum? Will the conflicts prevent use? Or, more probably, must the curriculum take some middle ground and, without compromising the expectations of the planners, cause the users to modify or at least put aside for the moment value positions which appear likely to arouse conflict?

Thirdly, we are not always certain of the source of our values. Do we value a certain nutrition-related concept because it has had some empirical justification? Do we value it because it has a cultural or social tradition? Do we value it because somehow it 'fits' with the way we view and make sense of the world? As curriculum planners we must be able to sort out these various modes of justification, of valuing, and be able to present them with reasonable precision to those who will be expected to use our curricula.

I have noted that curriculum planning is a form of social control
—most often institutionalized in places called schools. When the
notion of control is explicit rather than implicit, as is more often
the case, the importance of values becomes sharply apparent. We
must, as curriculum planners, develop the skill of rationalizing our
curriculum decisions, presenting that rationalization to those who
will engage themselves with our curricula, test the rationalization
against the values of our clients, and clarify for ourselves and for
others the bases for our valuing.

THREE CURRICULUM DESIGNS

With the understanding that the prior discussion regarding control
and values relates to all curriculum planning, I present three curriculum
designs for your consideration (Griffin and Light 1975). It should be
understood that each of these designs can be adapted or modified
to fit a particular socio-cultural milieu. Further, although the designs
are essentially different on certain dimensions, elements from each
might be shifted from one to the other so that some hybrid or
amalgam results which draws upon two or three of them to make a
fourth. What should be understood is that there is nothing sacred or
inviolate about any of the designs. They are ways of talking about
curriculum and curriculum planning—ways that have been seen to be
fairly productive and useful. What is important is that each of us, as
curriculum planners, considers which design or which recombination
of elements is most appropriate for the target population, for the
cultural surround into which it is to be placed, for the system of
values we start with, and for the problems which we wish to solve
or somehow ameliorate.

I have named the three curriculum designs: the rational–empirical
design, the engagements design, and the emergent design. These
labels are not ones commonly found in the curriculum literature—not
because I am arrogant enough to re-invent the wheel but because
they identify certain types of designs and therefore offer conceptual
frameworks which include specific designs by type. That is, when
one considers the rational–empirical design, for instance, one takes
into account that the work of various curriculum experts and theor-
eticians might be included under this rubric, but varying degrees of
specification and varying emphases would be present if one considered
the experts' work separately.

THE RATIONAL-EMPIRICAL DESIGN

The rational-empirical design is probably the most commonly used
and most widely known of the designs I will be discussing (Goodlad

1966). The design rests upon the assumption that school persons can and should plan in advance for what students will learn. The curriculem planner using this design has a responsibility to specify in the curriculum what shall be learned, how it shall be learned, how what is planned for shall be organized, and how what is learned is measured at the conclusion of an instructional sequence.

The most common form of specifying what shall be learned in the rational–empirical design is the behavioural objective. A behavioural objective is a statement which indicates the behaviour expected of students and the piece of content for which that behaviour is considered appropriate (Bloom 1956). It should be noted that the emphasis here is upon what the student is expected to achieve, not what the teacher is expected to do or what the school is expected to provide. Examples of behavioural objectives for nutrition education might include:

(1) to recall locally produced foods which provide high quality protein;
(2) to apply knowledge of the cultural milieu to the formulation of a community nutrition education programme;
(3) to demonstrate the relation of local food distribution systems to the presence of malnutrition in vulnerable groups;
(4) to formulate a plan to inform members of the community of the special nutritional requirements of various age groups; and
(5) to demonstrate the relation between local soil conditions and food which is or can be produced.

These examples illustrate that what is being presented in the objective for instruction is a combination of desired behaviour (recalling, applying, demonstrating, planning) and content (provision of high quality protein, the cultural milieu, community education programmes, food distribution systems, and so forth).

Once the objectives have been formulated it is the task of the curriculum planner in the rational–empirical design to present a set of learning opportunities which is believed to be powerful in achieving the desired ends. That is, what activities can be planned for students and teachers which can best accomplish the objectives? A problem with learning opportunity selection and formulation, especially in highly developed countries, is the prevalent dependence upon print. We require that people attend to books, texts, and so on, to a very large extent. We too often ignore the powerful possibilities of using activities which are essentially tactile, aural, manipulative, or a combination of all of the senses. Our dependence upon selections which are print-bound often limit the potential outcomes too rigorously. When we begin to expand the opportunities for learning beyond print we also expand the possibilities for learning. A balanced curriculum should provide opportunities for students to learn through reading, of course, but it should also include options which, for their success in achieving the behavioural objectives, call for students to touch and to manipulate and to construct and to analyse their environments through discussion. A critical issue and one which looms large as a criterion is the mode of learning most effective with a given population. Obviously to expect pre-school youngsters to read technical material is absurd. Equally absurd would be to expect older, more experienced and knowledgeable students to learn solely through the manipulation of physical properties. In formulating objectives and in planning activities to achieve them, we must attend to the particular learning characteristics and skills of our students. To do so is to include the student in our conscious planning—not just as the object of our work but as a data source to inform how we will go about our work.

The next major task for the curriculum planner in the rational-empirical design is the organization of the curricular elements. What is expected to be learned first? What sequence of activities is most likely to achieve the objectives most efficiently? What objectives are natural prerequisites for other objectives? The two concepts here are vertical organization and horizontal organization. Clearly vertical organization refers to sequence over time. What should happen first, next, last? What materials and activities are to be used with primary level students, with intermediate level students, with adult students? This vertical organization is a concept with which we are all familiar. Less obvious, however, is the concept of horizontal organization. This refers to those activities and objectives and other school-related phenomena which the student experiences at about the same point in time. As an example, we can consider the ten- or eleven-year-old student who, as part of his or her instructional sequence, participates in a nutrition education curriculum. That, much as some partisans might like it to be, is not his or her entire programme of studies. He or she is probably also studying mathematics, literature, some social sciences, physical education, and physical science. The notion of horizontal organization suggests that each of these bodies of knowledge and skill should, whenever possible, reinforce and build upon one another. A good integrated curriculum for our hypothetical student would attend to the relations between nutrition education, the humanities, and the sciences. What can the teacher of literature contribute to the understanding of nutrition concepts? What can the social science classes do to promote further understanding of a people's beliefs and mores as they relate to eating habits and customs? What can the science programme do to undergird with scientific principles the content of nutrition being taught to the student? Clearly there will be isolated learning present in any curriculum which, by their very natures, are not amenable to such cross-discipline treatment. But it is believed that acting out the concept of horizontal organization increases the power and the efficiency of the learning system.

Related directly to horizontal organization in the school is careful attendance to the experiences that students undergo in other, non-school parts of their lives. Most of us have other affiliations than that of the school. Students belong to organizations, social and civic. They are members of religious groups. They form *ad hoc* groups of peers. They are members of families. A systematic programme of instruction would pay particular attention to ways in which student activities in these non-school groups reinforce or are reinforced by the school programme. An example is the movement in the United States for both boys and girls to have experiences in food preparation and an understanding of the importance of nutrition to their lives. (Formerly only girls were provided with these opportunities.) A school which cares about the degree to which outside forces impinge upon school programmes would see to it that there is some food-related content in the local Boys' Club, that parents encourage participation in food preparation activities in the home, that summer jobs for students include ones related to food preparation or distribution, that church socials sponsor a boys' division in their food bazaars, and so forth. We must be conscious of the fact that the school provides considerably less than the student's entire education and, with that consciousness, we can intervene effectively with others so that our mutual concerns are attended to.

The final decision area facing the designer of a rational–empirical curriculum is that of evaluation (Bloom, Hastings, and Madaus 1971). Although this subject is treated in some depth and breadth by my colleague Professor Wolf I want to include it here because I fear that evaluation may sometimes be seen as being apart from curriculum planning. I neither believe that such is the case, nor that it should be. The curriculum planner who formulates behavioural objectives, plans learning opportunities for them to be accomplished by students, and organizes both into a coherent instructional sequence must also be concerned with how and under what circumstances it will be known whether the curriculum was effective or not.

Evaluation as I am talking about it is of two basic kinds: student evaluation and programme evaluation. We are most accustomed to student evaluation. We rate students with ease by giving them grades or percentage points or with some other system. The bases for these ratings, however, are often less easily articulated. What is it about a particular student that places him or her at the ninetieth percentile? What do we know about another to give him or her an A or a B or to award the coveted Honours rank? In the rational–empirical design, if we have formulated our behavioural objectives with precision and clarity, we almost automatically know what to look for in the student. If our objective calls for recall of certain principles and the student dutifully lists them, we know that he or she has achieved the goal. If we ask that students know how to plant and maintain a garden so that edible fruits and vegetables are the result, we can observe and examine the garden to see if, and to what degree, the student's behaviour matches our expectations of it. This is a very strong point in favour of this design—the direct and positive relation between the formulated objective and the evaluation process. But we must be careful, as planners, that our evaluation matches our objective. Too often we expect certain behaviours (or, at least, say we expect them) and then measure for other behaviours. The most common error here is one associated with the argument about the print-bound nature of instruction commented upon earlier. If we expect students to be able to manipulate and rearrange certain properties to produce something new or unique, we must insist that the evaluation processes call for that manipulation and rearrange-ment and do not depend solely upon a pencil-and-paper test. With pencil-and-paper instruments we are often testing for something beyond what we are teaching—reading and writing. Although reading and writing are, naturally, admirable skills for all students to possess, we are really more interested here in nutrition concepts and skills. We want to know if the student knows, understands, and cares about the nutrition principles and practices we think we are teaching. To depend only upon skill levels in reading and writing to find that out is to engage in poor evaluation practice and, more seriously, to do a disservice to students and to the teachers who work with them.

The second evaluation type is less familiar to us: programme evaluation. We sometimes ignore the fact that evaluation results, when they are disappointing, are often telling us something about our curriculum and instruction as well as something about our students. If we do not achieve our objectives with the level of ac-complishment we desire, we should re-examine our curriculum. Perhaps our objectives are unrealistic. Perhaps our learning oppor-tunities are not as appealing to students as we thought they were. Perhaps we have taught in an illogical sequence. Perhaps we have assumed that reinforcement from other areas was taking place when, in reality, it was not. Perhaps our evaluation procedures are not appropriate or are too highly technical for the students or, in some other way, poorly designed. When evaluation is conceived of as an opportunity for programme study and revision we can see that the curriculum planning process has come full circle. We revise or maintain or eliminate material according to information provided by students as they move through the curriculum. As we find that certain students do not learn, we reconceptualize what we expect or how we want to accomplish what we expect, or both. These programme decisions, then, take us back to the formulation of objectives, the provision of learning opportunities and their organization, and our methods of evaluation. If we are concerned about the relevance and about the effect of our curriculum designing we never allow this sequence to end but continue to edit, to modify, and to revise.

I began this discussion with the rational–empirical design because it suggests the elements to be manipulated in any design with some clarity. The other two designs will be presented more briefly.

THE ENGAGEMENTS DESIGN

The engagements curriculum design is one that depends largely upon the statement of values argued for earlier in this paper. In this design one sets forth a fairly elaborate statement of what is valued in a certain content or skill area and presents that which is valued for students' attention. Hence the term engagement: the student engages himself/herself with some valued skill, artefact, piece of knowledge, or activity. The selection of what the student is to become engaged with rests more upon the value placed upon the object of engagement than upon some idea of a predetermined outcome. The behavioural objective, therefore, has little or no place in this design. We expect students to learn from the engagements, though we do not specify in advance what that learning ought to be (MacDonald 1968).

Although this description sounds very primitive when so baldly stated, close examination indicates that this is the planning mode used most often by teachers and other school persons. When asked what a given class is doing or about, school people usually give answers such as, 'We're covering the protein content of fatty meats,' or 'The students are making models of molecules,' or 'We're trying to get through the materials on malnutrition by next Tuesday.' These examples give little or no attention to outcomes, or learning, by students. They do tell, however, what it is the students and the teachers are doing together. These conventional responses, though, are not indicative of a well-designed engagements curriculum because they are largely incomplete. A good engagement for students would be one which can be justified from a value position and which can be defended because it has a basic integrity unto itself. We assume that there is enough importance in having students interact with a certain piece of the culture for us not to need to preset what the students are to take from that instruction. An example might be the planting and growing of a garden. This school activity, common to most cultures, presupposes that growing a garden is a good thing. Naturally we expect that the garden will grow and be healthy and have some utility for us and for others but we do not suggest that understanding the phenomenon of growing is all that the students will get out of the activity. Some students may concentrate upon the properties of growth and will in effect learn some physical science as a consequence of the activity. Others may note the changing colours, patterns, and shapes that the plants assume and take aesthetic understanding with them as a consequence of gardening. Others may note the effect of water on soil and the relation between soil banks and water retention and consequently better understand principles and properties of soil conservation and environmental protection. The point is that we provide the activity because it is valued by the culture or by a powerful subculture and because we believe that students should have some understanding of that activity. Beyond these basic specifications, however, we allow the students to come away from the activity with what is most appealing, most intriguing, most meaningful to them.

This provision of opportunities to experience what a culture values, although less rigorous in terms of specification of outcomes than the rational empirical design, does not lack in rigour when it comes to the matter of evaluation. Evaluation of the engagements is the task of finding out whether or not the student attaches the same or similar value to the activity as the culture and, beyond that, what specific forms that value takes for each student. Evaluation here calls for the teacher or other person in charge of instruction to observe with precision to discover the degree to which the student attends to the activity, the responses elicited from the student by the activity, where the engagement leads the student as a consequence of his or her interest and needs, and so forth. These evaluation procedures, largely informal and much less highly structured than formal tests and such, call for a level of perception and a sensitivity to student responses that are as difficult to find as are examples of superbly designed standardized tests.

THE EMERGENT DESIGN

This curriculum design calls for the content and the nature of instruction to emerge from the concerns, needs, and desires of the students. Its most obvious manifestation is probably that of the British infant school and the subsequent open education movement that is now under some pressure from various interest groups. We have seen that the rational–empirical design is highly controlling in that the decisions about what shall be learned, how it shall be learned, how what shall be learned is organized and evaluated are all made pretty unilaterally by the curriculum planner. Less controlling is the engagements design, in that the consequences of the engagements are not decided precisely or in advance by the planner but still controlling in that the engagements are selected from a universe of possibilities by the planner (Griffin 1971).

In contrast to these designs, the emergent design is one that is controlled *by* students rather than controlling *of* students. One might think of this design as one in which the conventional relation of student and school is reversed. That is, the usual pattern is that the school is the stimulus and the student responds to that stimulus. We look for the degree to which the student responds appropriately to what we expect of him or her. In the emergent design the student is the stimulus. The school responds to what the student thinks or believes is necessary for his or her well-being. In such a design the school and the persons in it really do little in the way of specific planning for instruction. They do not prepare objectives. They attend only minimally to the pre-setting of engagements or activities. They instead develop a set of techniques and knowledges that will help them to clarify with students what it is that the students believe to be a desired school life. There is a tendency to look upon this mode of schooling as one which abrogates the responsibilities of teachers, one which has little or no structure, one in which the authority figures in the environment play little or no active part. Such is not the case. The skills necessary to eliciting from students what they think school should be about are formidably difficult to acquire. We school people are, in fact, much more skilful with, and accustomed to, telling and manipulating than we are in questioning and responding to students with sensitivity, awareness, and willingness.

In terms of nutrition education programmes, it is obvious that certain parameters must be set to contain what the school's responses and the elicitations of student expectations are to be. The limitation we would impose would be to specify that certain times in the day, or week, or term will be devoted to issues of nutrition and then to allow students to develop programmes of studies based on what it is that they want to know about or how to do. If this design were to be adopted it would be necessary for teachers and others in the school to have considerable understanding of the students in the programme, their cultural aspects as well as their cognitive and physical development stages. With such understanding of the students to be served by an emergent curriculum, one can anticipate what it is that students are likely to know already, what it is that they are likely to care about, what skills they are likely to be able to put to use, what questions or issues are likely to be intriguing to them, and so forth. The emergent design, more than either of the other two, calls for an intimate understanding of the client of the school's programme of studies.

In addition to the knowledge of the student, it is naturally incumbent upon the teacher and curriculum planner to have a ready and available understanding of the nutrition concepts and skills which are likely to be brought up for attention by the students. This understanding must be both broad and deep. It must contain information and behaviours that relate to knowledge of the students in that anticipated questions must be readily answered. The implication that the teacher must be all-knowing, however, is misleading. The teacher should naturally have command of the subject-matter but, perhaps more important, he or she must have command of the resources available to students which relate directly to the subject-matter. This command over resources is really the central role of the teacher in the emergent design. The teacher must be able to help the student wend his or her way through the often dazzling, sometimes confusing, mazes that constitute the growing body of nutrition science. The teacher, then, becomes a responder, a guide, a resource person, a questioner.

As in the other designs, the question of evaluation is one that must be addressed directly. To say that the students are the primary resources in the planning and execution of an instructional programme is not to say that the school does not have a major responsibility to judge how effective that instructional programme is or has been. As with the engagements design, the evaluation procedure draws little upon the notion of some pre-specified set of expected outcomes. Instead, the evaluation in the emergent curriculum focuses upon how effective the programme was in meeting the articulated needs and desires and questions of the students. Did what occurred as a consequence of student initiation really accomplish what the student wanted? Did the consequences appear to be reasonable to the student? To the teacher? To others in the school? To parents? What verification can be offered to justify both consequences and perceptions of consequences? What might the teacher have done to increase the power of the school experience for the student? What unanticipated outcomes were present as the instructional sequence proceeded? What expected patterns of behaviour on the part of students were observed? With what results? What unexpected patterns of behaviour emerged? With what results? These questions, it can be seen, are very different from those in either of the other designs.

CONCLUSION

This chapter has presented three curriculum designs. The designs are seen as three perspectives on the control of the matter of schooling—control over decision-making authority, the content and mode of instruction, the allocation of time and energy and other resources, and control over the outcomes of school programmes. The rational-empirical design, resting on the assumption that school persons and curriculum planners can and should specify in detail the expected consequences of schooling and the manner in which these consequences are induced, is seen as the most controlling. Somewhat less controlling is the engagements design which has as a central principle that certain encounters with the culture are intrinsically valuable and should be offered to students to deal with on their own terms. Least controlling is the emergent design which operates upon the reversal of the conventional schooling–student relationship —the school becomes the response mechanism and accommodates the stimuli presented to it by the students.

As was stated at the outset, the intention here is not to suggest that any of these designs is holy or in some other way sacrosanct. They are presented because they represent what are believed to be the three principal modes of thinking about and planning of curriculum. As one's cultural, social, political, and economic context is understood and acted upon appropriately, it is highly probably that elements drawn from each may be present in the resultant curriculum. It is important, though, to suggest that this mixing and matching be done with care, with thoughtfulness, with disciplined understanding of the nature of schooling within the society, and with constant attention paid to the effects of the implementation of the design upon students.

REFERENCES

Bloom, Benjamin (ed.) (1956). *Taxonomy of educational objectives: the classification of educational goals*. Handbook I. *Cognitive domain*. McKay, New York.
—, Hastings, Thomas, and Madaus, George (1971). *Handbook on formative and summative evaluation of student learning*. McGraw-Hill Book Company, New York.

Cremin, Lawrence A. (1977). *The education of the educating professions.* The American Association of Colleges for Teacher Education, Washington, DC.

Foshay, Arthur W. (1970). *Curriculum for the 70's: an agenda for invention.* National Education Association, Washington, DC.

Goodlad, John I. (1966). *The Development of a conceptual system for dealing with the problems of curriculum and instruction.* The University of California at Los Angeles.

Griffin, Gary A. (1971). *Schools for the 70's: a call to action.* National Education Association, Washington, DC.

— and Light, Louise (1975). *Nutrition education curricula: relevance, design, and the problems of change.* UNESCO Press, Paris.

Krathwohl, Davis (ed.) (1964). *Taxonomy of educational objectives: the classification of educational goals.* Handbook II *Affective domain.* McKay, New York.

MacDonald, James (1968). 'A curriculum rationale. In *Contemporary thought on public school reform.* Wm. C. Brown Publishers, Dubuque, Iowa.

Mager, R.F. (1962). *Preparing objectives for programmed instruction.* Fearon Press, San Franscisco.

Tyler, Louise and Klein, Frances (1971). *Preparing curriculum and instructional materials.* Tyl Press, Los Angeles.

Tyler, R.W. (1950). *Basic principles of curriculum and instruction.* University of Chicago Press, Chicago.

12 The implication of new approaches to learning for nutrition education

HOLGER HYBSCHMANN HANSEN

PSYCHOLOGY AND EDUCATION

Why should educationists—and people teaching nutrition—be interested in psychology? It can be noted that psychology is part of the training of most of the teachers, but surely this does not answer the question. In an attempt to answer this question I take as my point of departure *the teacher*. It should be stressed, however, that this word should be taken in its widest sense.

The pivotal link in the joint enterprise of creating a relevant and effective nutrition education is the teacher. The scientist in the laboratory must pass on his knowledge to the teacher, the educational researcher must convince the teacher of the relevance of his views, and so must the psychologist. This is why I aim directly at teachers when speaking of educational psychology.

Why then should a teacher be occupied with psychology? My answer is that the teacher is inevitably occupied with psychology. It is not possible for him not to be so. Like all human beings the teacher has some implicit psychological views that co-determine his relations to his fellow human beings and also to his pupils. Here I have in mind what Fritz Heider calls naive psychology (Heider 1958). What should be noted here is that this kind of psychology is not stated explicitly. The greater part of it may only be found by listening to what the teacher says or by watching his ways of teaching.

But why then should teachers be occupied with academic psychology? My answer is that psychologists may be of help to teachers if they can make the teacher aware of his own implicit ideas. The teacher's own ideas determine his actions, but if these ideas are implicit and nebulous his practice may become rigid and blind. In this situation the possibilities of profiting from experience is very limited. This vicious circle may be broken if the teacher can make his views explicit and compares them with the views of academic psychology. By making the ideas explicit they are made accessible for criticism from the person himself or from others.

This is easy to state in principle, but it is not so easy to carry out in practice. Academic psychology contains many different points of view and many unclarified concepts. But still: if there is the least chance of making better teachers through a co-operation between teachers and psychologists, this co-operation should be attempted. In this connection it is interesting to note that the view has been expressed that psychology itself may profit from it (Heckhausen 1976).

THE PSYCHOLOGICAL LEARNING CONCEPT AND EDUCATION

The concept of learning is a central one both in psychology and in education. It should not be forgotten, however, that the concept has different functions in the two branches of knowledge. In psychology —at least in American psychology—learning should be looked upon as a central concept in the attempt to build a general theory of behaviour. In education interest centres on human learning, and educationists are not only interested in describing learning in general terms. In education you try to describe learning in such a way that it is made possible to give prescriptions as to how to make learning happen. From a general point of view it is of interest to note that in learning how to ride a bicycle, to use a typewriter, to spell, and to extract the square root there is a common feature, the change in behaviour. The educationist cannot be satisfied with this general observation. In order to make the learning process take place as smoothly and effectively as possible he must base his actions on an adequate understanding of the processes that take place before this change in behaviour can be observed. And in this respect there are great differences between the four examples of learning.

An example of how an educationally relevant psychological description might look can take its point of departure in what a teacher can do. The Swiss professor Hans Aebli (Aebli 1976) does so in an interesting book, the title of which in English would be *Basic forms of instruction*. These basic forms are the following: telling, showing, or demonstrating; building up a sequence of actions; observing or examining; building up an operation; forming and using a concept; practising and repeating; testing, evaluating, and giving marks; and finally programmed instruction and the use of teaching machines.

As an example of how psychology is relevant, I shall summarize the psychological description of the first one.

THE PSYCHOLOGY OF TELLING

Social psychology is clearly relevant, as any educational situation fundamentally is a social one. There is a speaker and a listener, so you may use concepts as roles and expectancies. What goes on is *communication*. The medium used is predominantly linguistic, although there are a lot of contextual factors too.

The speaker wants to communicate some kind of subject-matter. This subject-matter can be conceived of in the form of images that can be built on perceptions through all sensory systems or on actions. Furthermore, the speaker uses certain concepts formed on the basis of perceptual images by abstracting certain features and combining them into some kind of cognitive category. Images of actions give rise to operations, that is highly abstract cognitive schemes of action.

These images, concepts, and operations are intimately connected with feelings and moods. Some of the things that the speaker has in mind have a special value for him, and therefore, you can see the speaker show positive and negative feelings and different kinds of emotion.

While emotions and values are not necessarily communicated through language, but through gestures, facial expressions, and so on, the subject-matter must be encoded in language. How shall we conceive of language? Chomsky has given a description of this and his theory has been most influential in modern psycholinguistics. (Chomsky 1968).

In the listener's mind you must picture the same cognitive structure. The decoding process involves the same psychological processes as in the above description, triggered off in a complementary manner.

PSYCHOLOGY IN EDUCATION: THE NEED FOR A COMPREHENSIVE VIEW

The example of the psychology of telling seems to me to reveal a need for a comprehensive view when trying to use psychology in an educational context. In the example you can find most of the fields covered by psychology: motivation, perception, and thinking, to name but three broad areas of psychological inquiry. What is more: when you try to understand one area you will find that you have to draw on the others. Perception is dependent on motivation and vice versa, there is an intimate connection between perception and thinking, and so on.

To complete the picture, place the system in an environment and add the time perspective. The person and his environment are mutually dependent on each other. A person cannot exist without an environment, and an environment only exists psychologically as perceived. We do not react to a physical environment *per se*, but to meanings. A profound understanding of psychology presupposes a historical and developmental perspective. Time perspective should also include the future.

NEW APPROACHES TO LEARNING

With this comprehensive view in mind let us have a look at what might be called new approaches to learning. In psychology as in education most 'new' ideas can be shown to have a long history. From the recent history of psychology I have chosen two headings that seem interesting to me in this connection.

The first one is cognitive psychology. Piaget and his theory of cognitive development and Chomsky's linguistic theory have presented a serious challenge to traditional American psychology. Partly as a consequence of this and partly because of dissatisfaction with the empiricist tradition, we have since the beginning of the sixties witnessed a new way of dealing with mental phenomena. Inspired by information theory and modern data-processing, an attack is launched on problems of perception, memory, language, thinking, and other processes underlying the intellectual side of human life. The build-up of the 'human cognizer' is often pictured in terms of a model frequently in the form of block diagrams and flow charts. Aebli's book has been mentioned already (Aebli 1976). Another outstanding book is Ausubel's volume (Ausubel 1968).

The second heading is Soviet psychology. This is new to most people in the West because of the problem of language. In the last fifteen to twenty years, however, several translations have been published. Vygotsky's (1962) classical volume *Thought and language* (which should have been translated as 'Thought and *speech*'), was one of the first ones. It contains ideas of great educational significance and deserves a close reading. Luria's investigations of the directive functions of speech deserve to be mentioned, and so do many other names which the reader can acquaint himself with by reading the volume by Cole and Maltzman (1969).

In this connection I should like to point out a theory that has received a lot of attention in the USSR and Eastern Europe since the fifties. It is the theory of one of Vygotsky's students, P.Y. Galperin on the development of mental acts. In this theory you can note several similarities with Vygotsky's theory, and it makes it especially interesting to educators that it is based on investigations of pupils in schools where they learned geometry, handwriting, arithmetic, history, etc.

Stated briefly, the theory shows how an external, concrete act through successive stages is internalized and becomes a mental act. In order to make it possible for the pupils to develop a mental act like performing substraction or using a scientific concept, the educator must find out how to present the subject-matter in a form that allows concrete, external action. Objects or representations of objects, like diagrams, outlines, models, or notes are necessary when starting the formation of a mental act. The very first step of the utmost importance, Galperin speaks of creating 'the orienting basis of an action'. The pupils should know as clearly as possible how their actions should be. Simply to let the pupils carry out the task by trial and error is deleterious.

From this first level, the formation of a mental act is carried out through the following steps or levels of fulfilment:

(1) acts based on material objects or materialized representations or signs;
(2) acts based on audible speech without direct support from objects;
(3) acts involving external speech to oneself; and
(4) acts involving internal speech.

At each level the act is generalized, that is, used on new material, abbreviated and greater mastery is shown in the increasing easiness and smoothness with which the act is performed. For relevant literature, see Galperin, Leontjew, *et al.* (1974) and Lompscher (1973).

SOME SELECTED TOPICS

Let me now indicate some conclusions based on these new approaches to learning concerning certain selected topics. I can only give some hints about a few, but the reader may consult the following two books for further information: Lesser (ed.): *Psychology and educational practice,* (1971) and R.M.W. Travers: *Educational Psychology. a scientific basis for education practice* (1973).

Language

Language is a key factor in all education. Investigations show that teachers use most of their time in the classroom talking to the pupils. This clearly points to a need for acquainting the teacher with psycholinguistic notions.

In Soviet psychology language is seen as the key factor in the formation of mental acts. Speech in the external form is internalized and becomes inner speech. In the end, after abbreviations and automatization, this inner speech occurs so rapidly that the person has an experience of imageless thought.

Piaget also acknowledges the importance of language but maintains that language can only be used fully in the stage of formal operations. Understanding of language presupposes an established cognitive structure. This does not mean that language should not be used, but that the teacher should use language as an accompaniment to actions. The understanding is built on the child's own actions.

Action

The necessity of action for real learning is stressed both by Piaget and Galperin. For Piaget actions with concrete materials are necessary for building images, concepts, and operations. For Galperin the starting-point of any formation of a mental act is concrete materialized action. But language is also necessary here, if only in the teacher's explanation of the task (task orientation).

Motivation

Neither Piaget nor Galperin is very explicit about this concept. Piaget's notion is akin to the notion of intrinsic motivation. For Piaget the use of an operational structure is rewarding in itself. It can be added that Heckhausen and Weiner (1972) have shown that motivational concepts should be described in terms of the person's own way of perceiving them. Motivation cannot be understood independently of the person.

Reinforcement

Reinforcement can be conceived of as information concerning results or as feedback. Rewards not specifically pertaining to the task may have unwanted side-effects. The principle of immediate reinforcement (behind, for instance, Skinner's programmed instruction) is not universally valid. Tasks involving motor responses which are not easily remembered need immediate feedback, while tasks easy to remember show no deleterious effect by delay. On the contrary, you may expect improvement by delay, presumably because of the rehearsal necessary for profiting from the feedback.

PSYCHOLOGY AND NUTRITION EDUCATION

I have maintained that educators cannot avoid using psychology, and that they may profit from making their implicit assumptions explicit, thereby making it possible to criticize them through a comparison with academic psychology. I have argued that it is necessary to take a comprehenisve view of psychology when trying to use it in an educational setting. It is not sufficient to use one psychological concept in isolation, e.g. the learning concept. But so far I have spoken only of education in general. How does Nutrition Education come into the picture?

First let me say that I am not sure that it is possible to point out specific implications from psychology for specific kinds of subject-matter. It is possible to point out some implications for education in general and it is a matter for further investigations to see how these implications work within the fields of different kinds of subject-matter.

Aebli's basic forms of instruction is an example of such general implications. Another more fundamental implication concerns what might be termed educational anthropology: how should we conceive of the basic nature of our pupil? Briefly stated the two approaches described above underline the necessity of looking at the person as involved in an active interaction with his environment. Instead of looking at him as an empty box handled with and filled by the environment, he is seen as an active agent, working on and changing the environment and thereby himself.

Secondly, I see nutrition education as a joint enterprise. I understand that nutrition itself is a joint enterprise, involving people from many scientific disciplines. Nutrition education makes it necessary to establish a collaboration, which brings me to my final point.

In this general context it has only been possible to state some basic points of view and to invite collaboration. It should not be forgotten, however, that for implications to work it is necessary to draw in concrete contexts pertaining to specific problems. It is necessary for the educator in nutrition to contact a psychologist—among others—to discuss the problems. Psychologists can be of use to educators by discussing questions like: What does it mean to learn this or that? How would people experience my actions? If I have succeeded in showing this I have achieved my goal.

REFERENCES

Aebli, Hans (1976). *Grundformen des Lehrens. Eine Allgemeine Didaktik auf kognitionspsychologischer Grundlage.* (9th edn). Ernst Klett Verlag, Stuffgart.

Ausubel, David P. (1968). *Educational psychology. a cognitive view.* Holt, Rinehart and Winston, Inc., New York.

Chomsky, Noam (1968). *Language and mind.* Harcourt, New York.

Cole, M. and Maltzman, I. (ed.) (1969). *A handbook of contemporary soviet psychology.* Basic Books, New York.

Galperin, Leontjew, *et al.* (1974). *Probleme der Lerntheorie.* (4th edn). Volk und Wissen, Berlin.

Heckhausen, Heinz (1976). Relevanz der Psychologie als Austausch zwischen naiver und wissenschaftlicher Verhaltenstheorie. *Psychol. Rdsch.* 28, 1–11.

Heckhausen, Heinz and Weiner, Bernard (1972). The emergence of a cognitive psychology of motivation. In *New horizons in psychology 2* (ed. P.C. Dodwell), pp. 126–47. Penguin Books, Harmondsworth.

Heider, Fritz (1958). *The psychology of interpersonal relations.* Wiley, New York.

Lesser, Gerald S. (ed.) (1971). *Psychology and educational practice.* Scott, Foresman and Co., Glenview, Illinois.

Lompscher, Joachim (ed.) (1973). *Sowjetische Beiträge zur Lerntheorie. Die Schule P.J. Galperins.* Pahl-Rugenstein Verlag, Köln.

Travers, Robert M.W. (1973). *Educational psychology. a scientific foundation for educational practice.* The Macmillan Company, New York.

Vygotsky, L.S. (1962). *Thought and language.* M.I.T. Press, Cambridge, Mass.

13 The role of evaluation in nutrition education

RICHARD WOLF

The role of evaluation in nutrition education can be stated quite simply: it is to improve the quality of nutrition education pro-grammes. As such it is an integral part of nutrition education rather than a peripheral enterprise undertaken to satisfy donor organizations or to produce impressive looking reports. Before proceeding to a consideration of some of the questions surrounding the evaluation of programmes in nutrition education, it is necessary to state what evaluation is and what it is not. It is also necessary to indicate, albeit briefly, what is involved in evaluating a nutrition-education programme.

Evaluation is defined as a deliberate and systematic effort to determine the worth of an intentional effort, whether it is an edu-cational enterprise, a social action programme, or some other helping effort. It involves the collection and analysis of five major classes of information. These classes of information are:

INITIAL STATUS OF THOSE WHO ARE TO BE SERVED BY THE PROGRAMME

Two kinds of information are required here. First, it is necessary to know who are the people to be served by the programme. What are their ages, sex, social background, previous educational history, etc.? Such information is necessary to describe adequately the group to be served. Secondly, it is necessary to know the initial status of such people with regard to what they are supposed to learn. Are they already proficient? If not, what is their initial degree of proficiency? Unless such baseline information is obtained, it will not be possible to estimate adequately the effect of the programme.

PROFICIENCY OF THOSE WHO ARE TO BE SERVED BY THE PROGRAMME AFTER A PERIOD OF TREATMENT

A programme of nutrition education is typically undertaken to bring about some changes in those who are to be served by the programme. Such changes could involve what people know, what they feel, and how they act. Any evaluation programme must systematically gather information about the extent to which these desired changes have occurred. Detailed information about such evidence-gathering and how it can be accomplished can be found in *A guide to evaluation of nutrition education programs* published by UNESCO.

EXECUTION OF THE PROGRAMME

Information about the way in which a nutrition education programme has been carried out is crucial. One can normally expect that there will be some discrepancy between a designed or intended programme and an actual or executed programme. If such discrepancies are small and arise out of the need to make some minor adjustments, then there is no problem. If, however, the programme that was carried out differs markedly from what was intended, then it is important to know this and the reasons for it. Failure to gather information about how faithfully the intended programme has been carried out can lead to the issuing of evaluative judgments about a programme that may be substantially different from what educators thought was being evaluated. This has happened far too frequently for comfort in the United States, for example. The only antidote is to make sure that the execution of the programme is examined so that one knows what is being evaluated.

COSTS

It is important to know how much an educational programme actually costs. A nutrition education programme that is tried out on an experimental basis could be so costly that no matter how effective it is in bringing about desired changes in people, large-scale implementation would be prohibitive. While educators often find it distasteful to consider the matter of costs in evaluating a programme, it is imperative that they do so.

There are a number of ways of reckoning how much a programme costs. Procedures range from basic accounting for only those additional costs that an institution actually incurs from having a particular programme (ignoring fixed institutional costs) to a cost-benefit analysis. This latter approach to cost determination is exceedingly complex and requires the use of highly skilled personnel. On the other hand the determination of additional costs needed to mount a particular nutrition education programme can be done rather easily by a person with elementary bookkeeping skills. The magnitude of the programme being evaluated will have considerable influence on the extent of a cost-reckoning operation. The important point is that some effort at costing be undertaken.

SUPPLEMENTAL INFORMATION

There are three sub-classes of information involved here. These are: first, opinions and reactions of various persons concerned with the programme being evaluated, secondly supplemental learnings; and thirdly side-effects of the programme. Opinion and reaction information about a nutrition education programme being evaluated can be critical. A programme, no matter how successful it is in achieving its goals, is likely to be short-lived unless it is accepted by learners, teachers, adminsitrators, and community groups. Accordingly information regarding the acceptance of the programme must be sought. It is conceivable that a well-intentioned programme may run up against local customs and taboos. If this is so, it needs to be known. An evaluation enterprise must make provisions for securing information regarding local acceptance of the programme.

Attempts should also be made to obtain information about what people are learning as a result of a nutrition education programme other than what was specifically intended. It may be that students are learning considerably more about nutrition than was intended by the programme. If this happy state of affairs exists, then it too should be known. Similarly if student attitudes are adversely affected by the programme this too should be known, even if attitude change was not a goal of the programme. Whatever effects can be made to secure information about things that people are learning in a programme other than what was specifically intended will add to the comprehensiveness of the evaluation.

The matter of side-effects of programmes is an elusive issue. We know from the history of pharmacology that drugs often have effects other than those that were intended. Identifying such effects is a difficult business, since one doesn't know what to look for. Educational programmes can have side-effects too. Follow-up studies are needed to identify what might be happening to persons who have gone through a particular nutrition education programme. Sensitivity, tenacity, and patience are essential ingredients for such work.

Once the five major classes of information outlined above have been gathered, it is necessary to analyse the resulting data both qualitatively and quantitatively to determine what is being evaluated, the effects it is having and the costs associated with the enterprise. The procedures for analysing data are generally well known and described in a number of standard textbooks. Once analysed, however, it is necessary to synthesize the results into a series of judgements about the worth of the programme and to make recommendation with regard to future action. The process by which this is done is not generally described in textbooks since it requires a set of carefully reasoned judgements on the part of those responsible for evaluation of the programme. There is, at present, some disagreement as to how judgements can and should be made. One must recognize, however, that the process is subjective in nature and cannot be handled by standard empirical methods and procedures.

There are a number of unresolved issues in evaluation on which debate continues. Some of them are presented below.

First, there is debate on how extensive the evaluation of a nutrition education programme should be. Technically-trained evaluation specialists are strongly inclined to restrict their evaluation to those cognitive learnings that can be readily assessed at the conclusion of a programme. The reason for this is very simple: it makes the job of the evaluation-specialist easier. This may not be acceptable to the nutrition educator who is seeking to produce effects that go beyond the programme itself. In fact, the nutrition educator may be principally interested in how people behave in their daily life after the programme has concluded. If this is the case, the evaluation worker will need to collect information from the field regarding out-of-programme behaviour. In addition, it will be necessary to find out what the competing influences are that the programme has to counteract. For example, there may be strong local customs operating on people in directions that are exactly opposite from those of the programme. Or, as in the case of the United States, there may be considerable persuasion in advertisements on TV and in other media that attempt to get people to behave in ways that are directly opposite to those being encouraged in the nutrition-education programme. In the area of nutrition education, it seems that the situation is extremely complex and will require efforts that go considerably beyond the boundaries of the customary teaching–learning situation. It should also be noted that programmes that aspire to have effects that transcend the classroom will need to develop learning experiences that also extend beyond the classroom.

A second issue on which there is considerable debate involves the use of comparison or contrast groups in evaluation studies. Stated succinctly, one group of evaluation specialists argues that the only effective way of determining programme effects is through the judicious use of comparison groups. The model for such work is the classic experimental laboratory study in which one group receives a treatment while another one does not. There are other evaluation specialists who maintain that not only are such elegancies unnecessary but unrealistic. Withholding a presumed benefit cannot be easily done. Setting aside the practical difficulties, there is still considerable question how necessary comparison groups are in many kinds of evaluation studies.

Finally, there is a fundamental debate surrounding the distinction between evaluation and research. This is reflected throughout the literature on research and evaluation. Some see evaluation as a special form of applied social research while others regard it as a separate and distinct enterprise. While this debate may seem foreign and academic to many, it has enormous implications for the design, conduct, analysis, and interpretation of results of evaluation studies. One such instance was noted above, the need for comparison groups in evaluation studies. There are other more far-reaching questions, such as how much confidence can one place in a programme that was tried and found to work in one location with one group of people? Will it work elsewhere if conditions differ? Must nutritional educational programmes always be particularistic or can one build a world-wide knowledge base about the field? In other words, is there something to be gained by having meetings such as this or must we stay within our own borders and try to work out local solutions to the problems of nutrition education as best we can? These are questions that urgently need to be asked and to have answers formulated.

14 The contribution of audio-visual techniques

MAX EGLY

This chapter presents a general approach to the subject and works from a practical viewpoint. It also presents a series of ideas in which the participants consider specific characteristics of audio-visual methods in the teaching of nutrition. Certain important points, connected either with the particular content of this teaching for certain groups or with the use of audio-visual methods as a means of diffusion of knowledge or a means of expression, are also considered.

Three points need to be made as general background.

First, the teaching of nutrition seems in general to be somewhat neglected in educational curricula. Even if in theory a limited place is assigned to it, there is no doubt that in practice this limited place is still further reduced.

Secondly, audio-visual experts are not usually concerned with questions pertaining to nutrition education. When these experts are interested in education they are more interested in literary, artistic, social, technical, or scientific fields when these have a visual aspect.

Thirdly, over the last two to three years there has been a noticeable fall in interest in the use of audio-visual techniques in education in general, and particularly in mass audio-visual education. This lack of interest comes from educationists as well as from decision-makers, administrators, or financial sponsors. Most frequently the effectiveness of audio-visual methods or their excessively high cost are the matters questioned.

These three preliminary findings might *a priori* seem discouraging. In fact, if one examines the different elements of the question, how best to use audio-visual methods in the teaching of nutrition, it becomes clear that there are still a large number of possibilities which have not yet been explored.

SOME GENERAL FACTS ABOUT AUDIO-VISUAL METHODS

We do not wish to dwell too long on the basic well-known characteristics of audio-visual methods but rather to recall some facts which are too often forgotten. A certain number of failures in the use of these methods is due to this. Examples which may be quoted are:

1. The category of audio-visual methods includes different types of equipment. These are extremely diverse in their potential for reaching the public, their costs, their flexibility in use, their suitability for instruction, and the number of persons needed to use them. For example, one cannot reasonably equate the use of a felt board with the national network of open-circuit television.

2. Certain generalizations which are always cited when speaking of audio-visual methods can only be justified when applied to certain methods. These include, 'a good sketch is better than a long speech', and, 'audio-visual methods allow one to reach the illiterate public in large numbers.'

3. The audio-visual method as an original means of expression and the audio-visual method as a wide-ranging means of diffusion of information should not be confused. The wide diffusion of an insipid or badly-structured document confers upon it no particular effectiveness.

4. One should beware of hasty judgements concerning certain audio-visual methods and the contents of their programmes. These generally lead to negative judgements such as, 'Radio cannot. . .', or, 'Television cannot. . .'. It is preferable to try to distinguish between specific types of radio programmes and television presentations.

5. Certain audio-visual methods have an instantaneous effect, for example when a diagram is shown on an overhead projector. Others work only when they act over a certain length of time, for example long radio or television series. One should therefore beware of limited experiments such as an isolated programme being shown to an experimental group and from this one programme drawing general conclusions about the series or, what is worse, about the medium itself.

6. The receptive public obviously plays a not insignificant role. For this reason one cannot speak in the absolute about the effectiveness of such-and-such a method. It will be much easier to teach nutrition to university students—a captive audience, motivated, and with a maximum of previous knowledge and a rich and sophisticated set of conceptual tools—than to mothers in a developing country—a free audience, unmotivated, lacking the indispensable informative and conceptual bases.

7. The elementary rule for any educational enterprise, 'to move from the known to the unknown', can equally well be applied when audio-visual techniques are being used. There one should beware of another dangerous misapprehension that 'audio-visual language is universal'.

8. When speaking of the effectiveness of an audio-visual method one should make clear the level at which one is thinking. The aim of the message can be:
    (a) to inform (that a certain food contains vitamins);
    (b) to make people understand (relating a certain illness to certain alimentary difficiencies);
    (c) to act on behaviour (leading the people to change their diet).
    It is important to take these various aims into account when an evaluation is undertaken.

9. Particularly where this last type of message (c) is concerned didactic audio-vision should not escape the elementary rule of all communication. This is to address the public as it is and not as one might wish it to be. Therefore one

should not neglect the important part which the irrational plays in human behaviour, as this directly determines the choice of themes treated and especially their presentation.

10. A permanent handicap must be pointed out. This is the scarcity of specialists in educational audio-visual methods. Although this field of activities has developed considerably over the last twenty-five years the real specialists in educational audio-visual methods are still very few and the conflicts between educationists, specialists in the particular content, and audio-visual artists continue. The problems are not, however, insoluble, and one can hope that a neo-professionalism will soon develop.

11. Finally it must not be forgotten that any audio-visual message can only be justified if it provides one or more specific elements and not if it is limited to reproducing an authorative lecture.

REMARKS ON SOME SPECIFIC ASPECTS OF NUTRITION EDUCATION

If the teaching of nutrition is considered only as a simple subject taking its place in formal education in the same way as geography or arithmetic then this teaching presents no particular problems as far as the use of audio-visual methods is concerned. If, on the other hand, the aim is to modify behaviour within the framework of formal education and if one is trying outside any educational institution to reach a part of the population other than school pupils a number of problems arise which invite us to reflect on the following points:

1. On the level of content: the teaching of nutrition relates to a certain number of ideas which are not immediately 'visualizable'. Like other creations of science, proteins, vitamins, and minerals are concepts which cannot be directly apprehended by any of the senses. Describing them will necessarily require a detour, a metaphor, or recourse to a more or less arbitrary code. A similar difficulty arises when it is a question of relating an illness and a food deficiency. The causality is far from being obvious and will demand a certain amount of imagination, and from the recipient a certain act of faith.

2. Particular obstacles must be pointed out. The teaching of nutrition does not deal with subjects from which the public can easily divorce itself. On the contrary it deals with food, which closely concerns everyone each day. The senses involved are taste, smell and touch. That is, precisely those senses which are absent from the audio-visual universe, and to express which audio-vision will have to find other methods of communication. Habits are questioned, habits so deep that they seem self-evident. It is well known how difficult it is to change eating habits, how difficult to overcome the force of unproven traditions, e.g. 'our grandparents all enjoyed never-failing health', or the tenacity of superstitions, 'alcohol makes you strong', or, 'to be overweight is a sign of prosperity'.

3. Certain difficulties present themselves frequently in whatever country the educational activity is being carried out and at whatever groups it is

being aimed. It is therefore most necessary that those who work in the audio-visual field consider certain subjects to be 'classics'. For example:

preservation of foods
parasitism
drinking water
presentation of a new food
environmental sanitation
enrichment of diets
evaluation of certain foods (e.g., as rich in proteins or vitamins).

4. For nearly thirty years educationists, doctors, scenario writers, and producers have brought a great variety of solutions to these classical problems. They have had to resolve problems of expression, such as the use of metaphors, real and abstract situations, and interviews. There are also problems of production for radio, cinema, and television and the presentation of major and minor themes within a series. There are also what might be called psychological problems of approach. For example is it more suitable to create a pessimistic documentary showing the horrors of illness or an optimistic documentary made up of pictures of happy life? Or, to put it more simply, does one consider health as the absence of illness or as positive well-being? Whereas the preparation of slides for secondary education poses only problems of readability and coherence of classification, the composition of a series of television programmes for a wide public raises particular difficulties. What tone should be adopted? Should it be serious and didactic or humorous? What concessions should one make to habits, e.g. can one transfer the virtues of the redness of Burgundy wine to the redness of tomato juice? Alternatively can one base one's approach on fashions? For example, the fact that older people commonly drink alcohol while young people drink milk. Or can it be based on snobbery where, in a developing country, the move from the maternal breast to the feeding bottle is a sign of modernity?

5. The most serious difficulty faced by the author of a document, the producer of a series of these, or the organizers of an audio-visual campaign is the danger of a 'boomerang effect'. This occurs when the effect obtained is radically different from the effect hoped for. The risk is particularly great when the teaching of nutrition is concerned. For example, a purely abstract demonstration runs the risk of not making the audience feel concerned, because they take the view that this is something which only happens in laboratories. On the other hand an excessively gloomy picture of an all-powerful and omnipresent microorganism risks generating fatalism on the principle 'We cannot do anything about it.' Equally an excessively humorous tone risks generating an off-hand reaction, with people thinking that the matter is basically not very serious if you can joke about it, while an excessively serious tone risks appearing to be moralizing, with viewers saying to themselves, 'They want us to feel guilty again.' And, of course, an excessively didactic tone runs the risk of suppressing all interest with its associations of a schoolroom.

LARGE- AND SMALL-SCALE EQUIPMENT

If, in practice, we want to indicate some useful directions for the undertaking of new enterprises we must establish a distinction between large-scale methods, which are aimed at very large audiences and require large investment, and small-scale methods, which are aimed at restricted, better defined groups of people and which can be used on limited financial budgets.

In general, whichever direction is chosen, a preliminary stage is necessary containing, as for any educational scheme, an identified goal and a preliminary grading of objectives, together with—and this is an important matter in the audio-visual field—information as complete as possible about the recipient public. In the case of developing countries such information is absolutely essential. It is only after these two steps have been taken that the choice of method can be made, taking into account the constraints—availability of funds, equipment, and specialized staff.

At the level of large-scale equipment we place the cinema, radio, and television, giving a privileged place to these last two media in so far as, used on open circuits, they are the most suitable for reaching an audience which is virtually unlimited, and for producing educational radio programmes. The criticisms levelled against the above media—diversity of the receiving public, centralization, and broadcasting at fixed hours—result less from an inherent weakness in the system than from the limited operations carried out in this way. They demand a great effort in planning, co-ordination, and control, and appeal less to individual producers than to small teams where educationists, doctors, and technicians work together. It is possible to measure, moreover, the best conditions for the effectiveness of these methods. Centralized broadcasting can include light but complete feedback, messages made directly accessible to the recipients, a high degree of repetition, linkage of a long series of programmes, group listening and viewing, and educational spectacle.

At the level of small-scale equipment we place all the auxiliary audio-visual apparatus, which is sometimes called the 'self-media'—pictures, slides, models, puppets, and sound and video recordings. These make possible the local production of documentaries and do not demand large financial resources nor recourse to a large team. This is particularly important within the school framework of a developing country where real decentralization is inevitable. The documentary is conceived and produced in the very place where the lesson will be given or the demonstration carried out. If necessary one specialist capable of acting as designer and photographer can do all that is required. Recourse to these 'self media' poses, however, a series of questions which need to be faced. These questions relate to the production of audio-visual presentations, to their back-up from written documents, and to the training of the staff who will use them.

15 The problems of instituting change in nutrition education

CY MAXWELL

It perhaps goes without saying that because the issue of innovation and change in education, with all its ramifications and implications for the system, for teachers, and for methods and materials, has been a major focal point, it has been the subject of considerable examination and investigation. There has consequently resulted a vast and increasingly scientific literature dealing with its various components and processes and the lessons which have emerged. Thus, it is perhaps also evident that a chapter of the scope of this one here would necessarily touch very briefly on numerous dimensions and aspects of the processes by which innovation and change are brought about. However, given that inevitability, it would perhaps be useful to review some of the basic dimensions of educational change in terms of roles, responsibilities, obstacles, and factors which may work both for an against innovation.

THE MEANING OF CHANGE

The terms 'educational change' and 'educational innovation' have been used more or less interchangeably. The distinction between the two, if indeed one exists, has usually been that by *change* one means alteration in a situation from one point of time to another and by *innovation* one means improvement of practices from one point of time to another. In all likelihood, such a distinction is rather artificial and unimportant in that whichever term may be applied, the process is aimed toward making a deliberate attempt to *improve* practices in relation to certain desired objectives, whether such attempts focus on altering and improving existing practices or introducing completely new methods and practices.

THE MANAGEMENT OF EDUCATIONAL CHANGE

We have noted that the terminology we have tended to apply when we talk of educational change has often involved words which if not interchangeable are at least seemingly overlapping. Thus, we talk of instituting change, managing change, implementing change. Perhaps, in the final analysis, again, these distinctions are not very important and we might do as well to settle on one, knowing that it may by implication mean at one time or another all three. However, because the Center for Educational Research and Innovation (CERI) elected to use 'management of change', I should like to use this term to denote the process by which change may be organized and instituted. In the present chapter, therefore, I should like to discuss briefly the concept of the management, the concept of educational change, problems in changing educational systems, and roles and functions in educational change. It perhaps goes without saying that the disucssion draws heavily from the work carried out by the CERI during its investigations into the management of educational change and which had been published in the OECD series 'Case Studies of Educational Innovation'.

THE CONCEPT OF MANAGEMENT

Increasingly pressures from a society in rapid change, changes in the student population itself, and in economy, technology, and attitudes have facilitated major changes in the educational institutions and systems, to the extent that no system today can avoid a careful and continuous search for better answers to increasingly pressing problems.

One would assume that a dynamic educational system necessarily would change the decision-making structure and concepts of management. This is not always the case, a phenomenon that can be observed in other organizations as well (e.g. industry). Instead of a rethinking of responsibilities, the existing power structure is effectively dealing with organizational and curricular changes through the use of management approaches and techniques that utilize research and development, planning and control techniques, and other more sophisticated strategies and tactics. In these systems, to manage change means the ability of the existing power structure to utilize the resources of the system while still maintaining the existing decision-making structure.

The management of educational change can no longer be looked upon as the domain of a few individuals, such as educational administrators, researchers, developers, or 'change agents'. The responsibility for change, its direction and the process, is a shared function among individuals and groups of students, teachers, institutional heads, researchers, administrators, politicians, and the public. It is a dynamic interplay of interests and forces among these individuals and groups that can facilitate a renewal process. The educational administrator will at any level of the educational system most probably have a particular responsibility as a facilitator and co-ordinator of the change process.

THE CONCEPT OF EDUCATIONAL CHANGE

As we have noted, educational innovation involves a deliberate attempt to improve practice in relation to certain desired objectives.

The underlying assumption in educational change, as we have defined it above, is that such changes, if successfully implemented, are useful and better than what they replace. The basic question, of course, is 'Better for whom?'. Since individuals and groups have different needs and differ in their goals, changes that concern several individuals and institutions will necessarily have different effects. For some, the results might be very positive. For others, the situation might be worse. And for many the changes do not matter. In understanding management problems in educational change it is of crucial importance to understand the various needs and goals of individuals and the most likely way in which the proposed changes will influence the lives of those involved.

PROBLEMS IN CHANGING EDUCATIONAL SYSTEMS

Any attempts to change a delicate and complex balance between goals, institutions, individuals, and programmes will have to cope with several types of barrier. In a practical situation it is often difficult to identify the type of barrier that is in operation. In many situations, several barriers are operating at the same time in an individual as well as in a group.

VALUE BARRIERS

People have different values. Some might understand these as differences in social and economic interest and others again will explain them as basic, intrinsic values, arising from varying relationships to the culture. Most significant educational innovations do face the problem of value differences. They are clearly apparent in changes such as moves towards racial integration, integration of disadvantaged in the normal school, introduction of sex education, changes from clear authority structures to participatory systems, and in changes that implicitly alter the relationship between education and society. Value conflicts are less apparent in innovations in subject-oriented matters (e.g. modern mathematics) and in innovations concerning the administration and organization of the system. If one studies some of the problems that these innovations face, however, value conflicts are also apparent as well.

POWER BARRIERS

Significant innovations usually mean a redistribution of resources and changes of authority structures in the system. Major educational reforms also tend to change the relationship between the educational system and other sub-systems in society (e.g. social services, the church). There are examples of innovations where individuals and groups volunteer to reduce their power for the benefit of others. These situations are rare, since most individuals and groups tend to hold on to their power, which very often means privileges and advantages that would otherwise be lost.

PRACTICAL BARRIERS

It has been said that most innovations fail because they are not good enough. We do not know if this statement can be verified, but many barriers can be traced back to either the characteristics of the innovation itself, or the institutional context in which it is developed, or the system context or the 'environment' (society context) in which it has to survive.

Many innovations break down in the dissemination and implementation phase, because the incentive structure of the system does not encourage innovative behaviour. In fact, such behaviour is punished by extra loads of work, uncertainties about outcome, scepticism among colleagues, and lack of support from external resources. Since the system is designed for maintenance, innovations will run into a number of practical barriers because of existing laws, regulations, examinations, and other control mechanisms. It is necessary for an innovation to survive to build 'shelter conditions' that protect the innovation from surrounding control mechanisms.

One of the CERI case studies indicates that a school can change its practices if it does not change the function of the school as understood by parents and society at large. Certain cases illustrate that when, for example, external control measures, like examinations, are removed from particular innovative schools to enable teachers to change the curriculum according to their innovative ideas, other control mechanisms, sometimes initiated by the parents, are set up to control the school. Many innovations face a number of practical barriers, either due to the lack of understanding of the relationship between the school and the environment, or because of inadequate mechanisms to deal with those conflicts that will arise.

PSYCHOLOGICAL BARRIERS

Many strategies for change are used to lower the resistance to change or to overcome barriers. Some of the research regards resistance as something unwanted and a personality trait more than anything else. Social engineering techniques and related strategies have sometimes been used uncritically to overcome resistance.

Analyses by psychologists and social psychologists, among others, indicate that people tend to continue with activities that are known and have a certain security, rather than go into activities with unknown consequences. Self distrust, insecurity and regression, and dependency on authority figures have also sometimes conservative effects. There are many patterns of behaviour that can support personality resistance. In most cases, the innovations are rejected either through ignorance, by maintaining the *status quo* by following the norms of influential, interpersonal relations or by creating substitutes.

FACILITATING FACTORS IN CHANGE

There are, of course, a number of positive factors in any change process. If there were no facilitating forces a successful implementation of change would be impossible. Usually a whole range of facilitating forces can be taken into account.

Political forces

Major changes usually have the support of certain political parties or interest groups. What is called 'political' will differ from case to case and country to country. Support for a particular innovation usually comes from individuals and groups with similar social-economic interests and with common values and beliefs, or both.

Management capacity

Even if the ordinary administration usually has little capacity left for rethinking and innovative practices, most systems have created planning units and innovative agencies that can push significant innovations, at least at the planning and development stage. It is increasingly accepted in most countries that both the state and the local administration will have to play a leadership role in educational change. A rethinking of the decision-making structure, including the question of centralization or decentralization, changes in roles and functions in the system, can provide unique opportunities for change.

Resources

Although resources might be a crucial problem, most major change efforts will get some additional resources for the initial costs connected with the development work. Over the last years educational institutions in Member countries have been increasingly facing resource problems. Undoubtedly this is a factor that might influence educational change considerably but not necessarily halt such efforts or make educational changes less 'useful' or 'relevant'. Among other things, an analysis of the allocation of resources has illustrated the potentials in reallocations and the use of new incentives geared to new innovative objectives and practices.

Human resources

A major change effort will always attract a core group of teachers, heads, administrators, researchers, and others, who will be devoted to the development of the idea. High motivation and enthusiasm is often necessary in the hard and difficult task of starting a change effort. A change in roles, for example the change in the role of the inspector towards a consultative role in change, sometimes connected with regional development centres, changes the relationship between school and administration and has potential for the support of educational change. In some countries, but only in very few, additional consultancy capacity exists for planning, evaluation, organizational development, leadership training, and other specialized skills which can support educational change. A flexible use of such additional resources is an important facilitating force in change. Most research on change shows the importance of leadership. It is probably true that few innovations would have been initiated without the energy, courage, and skills of one or a few individuals. Throughout the life of an innovation leaders might change, so will the need for different leadership skills, but no doubt leadership is a necessary resource.

ROLES AND FUNCTIONS IN EDUCATIONAL CHANGE

Any major educational change, like any social change, means changes at the level of the individual, the institution, the system, and indeed the society, involving many individuals and groups. It might imply that behaviour changes are necessary, but, more important, in certain cases opportunities will be altered, the school as a working place will change its character and climate and basic human relationships might change. This is why the question of *who decides what*, and in what context I as a participant in a system in change am involved, is of crucial importance. Much research indicates that both the direction of change (where are we aiming?) and the quality of the process are dependent upon who is basically involved in key positions and groups. This is true for the students and teachers, administration, researchers, other support personnel, politicians, public, and indeed the parents.

There appear to be two main trends in the development of roles and functions in educational change:

1. The old roles of administrators, inspectors, teachers, students, and parents
    are slowly altered, but the basic decision-making hierarchy is maintained. In
    addition, new roles are added to the old ones as support functions in the
    process, such as people in research and development institutions, production
    units, liaison people ('change agents'), and consultants. If one looks at the
    various educational systems in Western Europe and North America, one
    sees that this is the basic trend. There are considerable differences in the
    extent to which additional roles and functions are added to the process, in
    part dependent upon the degree of centralization or decentralization in the
    system. The emerging structure is thus a reflection of traditional patterns,
    with various additions as a reaction to crisis and *ad hoc* arrangements.

2. The other alternative is based on a radical rethinking of roles and responsi-
    bilities in the change process. It is not only a question of centralization or
    decentralization of authority but rather who should be involved in what
    type of decisions at what stage of the process of change. There is obviously
    no one structure that is feasible for all countries. Several factors, such as
    tradition, culture, and political, economic, and social structures and the
    relative role education plays in a given society are parameters of great
    importance in proposing a structure that can cope with an educational
    system in change. Certain critical issues, however, need to be taken into
    account in all countries.

    These include the type of innovation, the existing decision-making
    structures, and the available resources. All these are important but can only
    be mentioned here as matters which require consideration. Naturally there
    are also important role-relationships to be considered in the educational
    hierarchy, ranging from the politician who is involved in Government
    policy-making to the paid consultant who is brought in for his specialist
    knowledge. Inevitably, too, the students are involved both in participation
    of defining educational change and in implementing innovations. An active
    participatory role implies in the long run a redefinition of responsibilities.

16 The impact of malnutrition on the learning situation

SVEN AMCOFF

Malnutrition can be defined as the lack of a sufficient quantity or quality of nutrients to maintain the body system at some definable level of functioning. It has been estimated that 37–80 per cent of all pre-school children in the developing countries suffer from protein-calorie malnutrition as assessed by the manifestation of syndromes, nutritional indexes, and weight deviations (Bengoa 1974). Mild to moderate malnutrition, also called chronic undernutrition, is much more common than severe forms, and is often difficult to recognize. The severe forms are either due to insufficient protein and calories (marasmus) or to an acute protein loss or deprivation (kwashiorkor). The consequences are somewhat different, but obviously there is a continuum between normality, marasmus, and kwashiorkor. In this short article it is not possible to go into details, and the term 'mal-nutrition' will be used in a broad sense. The consequences of early malnutrition depend on a complex pattern of factors such as its severity and timing (pre- and/or post-natal) and the psycho-social milieu.

Today when increasing investment is being made in educational programmes in the developing countries, it is especially important to study the effects of early malnutrition on the ability of children to profit from education. Does early malnutrition impair the learning ability and school performance? If it does, is the effect permanent or can it be reversed with adequate nutrition? Is the education of malnourished children meaningless, unless they are simultaneously provided with proper food? These are some of the questions I will discuss.

MALNUTRITION AND SCHOOL PERFORMANCE

Unfortunately very few studies have been made concerning the direct effect of early malnutrition on school performance. The findings in those that have been carried out indicate that both chronic under-nutrition and severe clinical malnutrition in childhood are related to scholastic backwardness (Tizard 1974; Richardson, Birch, Grabie, and Yoder 1972).

There have been many investigations, however, regarding the

effects of early malnutrition on variables that might be expected to be of significance for school performance.

From the beginning of the 1960s knowledge has accumulated about the way that different types of undernutrition, occurring during different phases of development and at varying times, have influenced the development of the central nervous system in animals. It has also been documented for a long time that the cognitive development is delayed in children who have suffered a serious lack of nutrition for a considerable length of time. Attempts have been made to correlate these findings, and—in somewhat simplified terms —it may be said that undernutrition in the foetus and young child causes disturbances in the morphological and functional development of the central nervous system. These in turn affect the cognitive and emotional development of the child. On the other hand, behaviour scientists have shown how an unstimulating society and psychological environment delays and disturbs a child's development. When under-nutrition occurs, such an environment is almost always found, and to establish the existence of a causal relationship between undernutrition alone and cognitive development is very difficult. In the following I shall try to elucidate briefly the importance of good balance between adequate nutrition and a socially and psychologically stimulating environment for a normal development.

I shall deal firstly with biological effects of undernutrition and secondly with the way in which it is believed that these effects influence behaviour.

BRAIN DEVELOPMENT

If we first look at the effect of malnutrition on the central nervous system we find that a great deal of research has been done on animals but also that an increasing number of studies have been based on humans. In the former it has been shown that during periods when the brain is growing rapidly it is particularly sensitive to insult. This critical period theory has been applied to man, and as the neural cells multiply in the foetus during pregnancy, malnutrition of the pregnant woman can be dangerous to the foetus. But this critical-period theory seems to be too simple and is not easily proved in humans. It is complicated by the fact that different parts of the brain have their growth spurt during different periods, the time of which is difficult to settle. Thus damage occurring at one particular period will affect one part of the brain more than another. To make things even more difficult these periods differ between different animals and between animals and man. Generalizations from animal research to man thus cannot be made with certainty.

The parameters that have been used to indicate brain growth include the total number of cells (neurons and glia cells), the proportion of cells in different parts of the brain, myelin formation, cell size, axon–dendrite connections, and certain biochemical processes. There may also be other indices that have not yet been considered.

Pre- and post-natal malnutrition has been shown to affect all these parameters. The pre-natal multiplication of neural cells mentioned above is considered most important because these cells, which form the functioning cells of the nervous system, do not multiply after birth. The glia cells are also pre-natal in multiplication, but they form connective tissue in the nervous system and may not be so vital. Stein and Susser (1976) recently argued that during the second trimester of pregnancy when neurons multiply rapidly, the nutritional needs of the foetus may be small enough for the mother to sustain under any conditions that support her own life. The third trimester is the phase of maximum brain growth and also the period when foetal growth is most sensitive to nutritional deprivation, but it may not be the period when the most critical brain development occurs. Hence the foetus may be protected from irreversible damage to the nervous system and cell growth can take place post-natally. Recent research has also shown what rapid brain growth may persist into the second year of life or even longer. It is now supposed that a combination of pre- and post-natal malnutrition is necessary for irreversible damage to occur. There is still a lot of confusion concerning this question, however, and very little seems to be known about the long-term effect of rehabilitation during different post-natal periods on the various brain parameters.

BEHAVIOURAL DISTURBANCES

Certain behavioural alterations are found in malnourished children. In his review of the knowledge concerning the impact of severe and moderate malnutrition on behaviour, Read (1973) finds that severe malnutrition during pre-natal life or infancy or both is accompanied by apathy, irritability, maladaptation in social situations, a low attention-span and reduced exploratory behaviour. Other changes in behaviour that have been reported to be associated with severe early malnutrition are hyperexcitability to aversive stimuli and phobic reactions instead of normal curiosity toward new objects (Barnes 1971), as well as a decreased ability to focus on tasks and an increased emotionality (Thorp 1975). The behavioural disturbances found in hungry and moderately undernourished children include listlessness, apathy, and a lack of interest in the environment (Read 1973), as well as restlessness and a reduced ability to pay attention (Liggo 1969).

These behavioural disturbances most certainly interfere with learning. In order to learn and perform well at school the student must be active, attentive, curious, and explorative. He must also be able to focus on tasks and cope properly with social situations. These demands are poorly met by malnourished children.

MENTAL DEVELOPMENT

Now it might be asked 'What are the relations between the brain parameters and mental development or intelligence?' So far, it has unfortunately been as impossible to establish any relationship between brain cell number and intelligence as to relate intelligence to chemical processes (Dobbing and Smart 1974).

But we know that early severe malnutrition is related to retardation in mental development, as measured by different psychological tests. The intelligence of malnourished children has been found to be significantly lower than that of normal children. Language retardation is particularly evident in previously severely malnourished children. Cravioto (1970) emphasizes, however, that since psychological tests are not culture-free, a better measurement of mental development is the ability for intersensory integration of the central nervous system. The results of his studies (Cravioto, Gaona, and Birch 1967) show that malnourished children have delayed development of the ability to integrate auditory and visual stimuli as well as visual and kinesthetic stimuli. This is probably not only a perceptual process but also a conceptual one, where language is involved. Pollit and Thomson (1977) have recently made a critical review of studies on the effect of protein-calorie malnutrition on mental development. They conclude that 'except for those cases of severe and chronic undernutrition with an onset during the prenatal period or early postnatal life, protein-calorie deficiency does not *arrest* development'. But they stress the fact that in areas where malnutrition is endemic the social and psychological milieu is unstimulating, which also affects cognitive variables.

The abilities mentioned above are of great importance in learning situations. Language is the instrument by which new concepts are learned, as well as being the means of communication, the transmission of knowledge, thought, and the expression of thought. Language retardation is therefore a serious handicap at school and has a close impact on the ability to learn, to read, and to write. And visual–kinaesthetic intersensory integration is of great importance in learning to write. Consequently, delayed development in these areas predisposes to school failure.

LEARNING ABILITY

A more direct study of the learning ability of malnourished children has been made at the Tulane University Early Childhood Research Center in New Orleans ('Hungry children lag in learning' 1971). Learning ability was measured by practical learning tests, and a significant relationship was found between malnutrition and impaired learning ability. It is proposed that the difficulties of the malnourished children in maintaining attentiveness may be the key factor underlying the results.

INTERACTION BETWEEN EARLY ENVIRONMENT AND EARLY MALNUTRITION

Thus, early malnutrition is associated with abnormalities in brain development, behavioural disturbances, mental retardation (as measured by IQ tests or tests of intersensory integration), and impaired learning ability. There is no evidence, however, that early malnutrition is the direct cause of these disturbances (Barnes 1969) except in certain severe cases (Thomson and Pollit 1977). Malnutrition is generally found in poverty areas where there is also serious deprivation of environmental stimulation, a condition that could *per se* cause poor psychological development. To determine whether a causal relationship exists between two variables (in this case early malnutrition and mental disturbances), and not merely an association, the investigation must be designed as an experiment with controls. For ethical reasons this is not possible in the study of early malnutrition in humans. The researcher is thus restricted to survey studies or animal experiments, the results of which cannot be directly extrapolated to humans.

But sometimes such investigations can be made. The Dutch famine of 1944-5 in the Second World War is an example. Data from this situation have been treated as if an experiment had been performed. Large groups of children suffered this famine during different stages of development. The famine lasted from October 1944 to May 1945 and the effect has been carefully investigated by Stein and Susser (1976). They concluded, using data from the famine and from later examination for military service, that no relationship could be established between poor pre-natal nutrition and mental competence.

In developing countries where malnutrition occurs during both pre- and post-natal periods, the conclusion drawn by many scientists (Pollit 1970; Cravioto 1970, and others) is that the impairments are probably caused by malnutrition in complex combination with other factors found in poverty areas, e.g. socio-economic factors such as deprivation of environmental, social, and emotional stimulation, cultural factors, such as ignorance and illiteracy of the parents, and biological factors, such as infections (caused by poor hygiene), multiparity, closely spaced pregnancies, and prematurity. Cravioto (1970) presents several series of flow diagrams showing possible interrelations among these factors.

ARE THE EFFECTS PERMANENT OR REVERSIBLE?

As to the permanency of the effects of malnutrition, there seems to be a critical dividing-line at 6 months of age. In children who were less than 6 months when malnourished, changes in the central nervous system, mental retardation, and the impairment of the learning ability have been found to be permanent, whereas re-feeding has resulted in recovery in all these areas in children who were older than 6 months at the time of malnutrition (Winick and Rosso 1974). Both enrichment of the environment and provision of food lead to an improvement in mental performance in these children. But the data on this matter are far from sufficient to draw definite conclusions.

PROGRAMMES FOR COMBATING MALNUTRITION IN
YOUNG CHILDREN

Several studies have shown that in order to greatly improve the psychological behaviour and learning abilities of malnourished children, *both* better nutrition and stimulation for education must be provided (Read 1969). In a report on a Mexican study, Chavez, Martinez, and Yaschine (1975) described how supplements to the diet of the mother–child dyad had a positive effect on the child's behaviour and how, as a result, the child received more attention not only from its mother but also from other family members. The children slept less, played more, and were also more demanding and disobedient, all of which contributed to a normal development.

Freeman, Klein, Kagan, and Yarbrough (1977) also report successful results of a nutrition intervention programme in rural Guatemala. They stress that such programmes are relatively easy to implement in comparison with most other social action efforts, but they limit their conclusions to the area studied, probably being aware of the possible influence of cultural habits and factors in the environment.

In a recent article by Guthrie, Masangkay, and Guthrie (1977) the social aspects of malnutrition are stressed. They have worked in Sagada Mountain Province in the Phillipines and have studied a group of severely malnourished children. The children were breast-fed during the first critical six months of life and had thus received adequate nutrition during that time, but during the post-weaning period they did not receive sufficient nutrients, partly due to the fact that they suffered from diarrhoea.

The authors stress, however, the constraints of the cultural milieu, which, via the parents, teaches the children a pattern of passive resistance. This leads not only to resistance to nutritious foods when offered, but also to cessation of activities and refusal to respond to others. The result is a child cut off from what he needs for both cognitive development and physical growth.

CONCLUSION

It is evident that malnutrition and its consequences are determined by a complex pattern of factors. This should be kept in mind when planning intervention programmes, and consideration should be paid not only to the supply of nutrition but also to improvement of socio-psychological conditions. The importance of a satisfactory balance between nutrition and a stimulating environment increases, however, with the age of the child, the need for adequate nutrition predominating in the pre-natal and early post-natal period. As the child grows, his mental development is perhaps more dependent upon the social environment than upon adequate nutrition. Before any definite conclusion can be drawn, however, about the relative long-term effects of supplementary nutrition and socio-psychological stimulation, and thus of the benefits of intervention programmes, further research in this field must be undertaken.

REFERENCES

Barnes, R.H. (1969). Effects of malnutrition on mental development. Truths and half-truths. *J. home Econ.* **61**(9), 671–6.
— (1971). Nutrition and man's intellect and behaviour. *Fed. Proc.* **30**(4), 1429–33.
Bengoa, J.M. (1974). The problem of malnutrition. *WHO Chron.* **28**, 3–7.
Chavez, A., Martinez, C., and Yaschine, T. (1975). Nutrition, behavioural development and mother–child interaction in young rural children. *Fed. Proc.* **34**, 1574–82.
Cravioto, J. (1970). Complexity of factors involved in protein-calorie malnutrition. *Bibl. 'Nutr. Diet.'* 14, 7–22.
— Gaona, C.E., and Birch, H.G. (1967). Early malnutrition and auditory-visual integration in school-age children, *J. Spec. Educ.* 2(1), 75–82.
Dobbing, J. and Smart, J.L. (1974). Vulnerability of developing brain. *Br. Med. Bull.* 30, 164–8.
Freeman, H.E., Klein, R.E., Kagan, J., and Yarbrough, C. (1977) Relations between nutrition and cognition in rural Guatemala. *Am. J. Publ. Hlth,* **67**, no. 3, 233–9.
Guthrie, G.M., Masangkay, Z., and Guthrie, H.A. (1977). Behaviour malnutrition and mental development. *Ekistics,* 43, no. 255, 74–6.
Liggio, F. (1969). Interference in the performance of the mental activities due to the wrong diet which lacks the protein factor on animal origin and nervous disorders which are complementary and reversible. *Acta neurol.* July, 24(4), 548–56.

Pollitt, E. (1970). Poverty and malnutrition: Cumulative effects on intellectual development. *Les Carnets de l'enfance*, 14, 40–9.
— and Thomson, C. (1977). In *Nutrition and the brain* (Vol. 2) (ed. R.J. Wurtman and J.J. Wurtman). Raven Press, New York.
Read, M.S. (1969). Malnutrition and learning. *J. Am. Educ.* Dec., 11–14.
— (1973). Malnutrition, hunger and behaviour. I. Malnutrition and learning. *J. diet. Ass.* 63, 379–85.
Richardson, S.A., Birch, H.G., Grabie, E., and Yoder, K. (1972). The behaviour of children in school who were severely malnourished in the first two years of life. *J. Hlth. & Soc. Behav.* 13(3), 276–84.
Stein, Z.A. and Susser, M.W. (1976). In *Malnutrition and intellectual development* (ed. J.D. Lloyd-Still), p. 39. MRP Press Ltd, Edinburgh.
Thomson, C.A. and Pollitt, E. (1977). In *Malnutrition, behaviour and social organization* (ed. L.S. Greene), p. 19. Academic Press, New York.
Thorp, F.K. (1975). A report of a presentation regarding learning disabilities from nutritional and learning points of view. *Journal of the Association for the Study of Perception* 10(1), 39–40.
Tizard, J. (1974). Early malnutrition, growth and mental development in man. *Br. med. Bull.* 30(2), 169–74.
Tulane University Early Childhood Research Center (1971). Hungry children lag in learning. *Opportunity* 1(3), 10–13.
Winick, M. and Rosso, P. (1974). In *Early malnutrition and mental development* (ed. J. Cravioto, L. Hambreus, and B. Valquist), p. 61. Almqvist & Wiksell, Uppsala.

Section III
Nutrition education in practice

17 Observations on the UNESCO report on the survey of the position of nutrition within the educational system

FRANCIS L. BARTELS

As one of its activities in the encouragement and improvement of nutrition education programmes throughout the world UNESCO in 1976, in collaboration with the International Union of Nutritional Sciences (IUNS), undertook a survey of the position of nutrition education within educational systems in its 135 member states. Questionnaires were formulated and distributed to gather information about (1) policies and planning for nutrition education programmes, (2) the development of curricula, (3) organization, methodology, and resources currently used in teaching nutrition, (4) the training of educational personnel, and (5) the institutional facilities and financing relative to nutrition education.

In a covering letter accompanying each questionnaire, the anticipated outcomes of the study were stated as follows:

> The results of the study should enable UNESCO and the IUNS to:
> (a) formulate recommendations for the integration and coordination of nutrition into the general education requirements of a country;
> (b) provide participating countries with more information, research material and experience, with which to adapt and further develop nutrition curricula in contemporary, changing societies; and
> (c) assist participating countries in drawing up guidelines and plans in the field of nutrition education, and to foresee the means for their execution.

With these goals in mind, it was suggested that each country involve a variety of people—educators, nutritionists, members of the Ministry of Education, etc.—in discussing each question and in formulating replies so that the final completed questionnaires would reflect a national consensus.

In April 1977 Helene Gordon and Doris Calloway of the University of California at Berkeley presented the results of extensive analyses of 60 questionnaires received up to that time (Gordon and Calloway 1977). The report document was 126 pages long plus appendices. There were 41 tables and 18 illustrative charts included, along with the written summaries of findings from the regions: Africa, Arab States, Asia, Latin America and the Caribbean, Europe and North America. Even within one region the countries were diversified in many factors, so that, as would be expected, answers were diversified, but certain findings were general and classification was possible.

After this impressive report was completed, additional question-naires were received by UNESCO from nine countries.

This chapter uses some of the data, summaries, and tables presented in the Report of the Survey as a basis for a number of conclusions and observations and observations on experience, mainly at the pre-university levels of education and in teacher-training, which are relevant to the less developed countries of the world in general and to Africa in particular. That it does not single out the position in higher education for the special mention it deserves is due in part to a recognition that the developing countries are becoming in-creasingly aware of the importance of a fourth dimension—service to the community—to higher education's traditional threefold mission of teaching, training, and research, and that awareness establishes nutrition education as a function of all four dimensions, requiring no elaboration in a general paper of this kind.

It is realized that conclusions drawn from a report based mainly on answers to questions addressed to governments may raise certain questions. The first is how much objectivity can reasonably be expected from all national governmental authorities in an evaluation process which in the final analysis must become an exercise in self-assessment for public consumption. The second is whether the purpose of certain questions have been interpreted differently in different countries, and the third is to what extent the meaning and significance of the same word might differ with different authorities. Finally, there is the question of how the role of the public and parents in a predominantly pre-literate community, for example in Africa, would be assessed. Although these questions limit the general-izations which can be drawn from the responses to the questionnaire, they do not invalidate the findings of the Report, especially as the International Union for Nutritional Sciences collaborated, to the greatest extent possible, with government authorities in maintaining a desirable level of technical appraisal.

This paper is arranged in three parts. Part I is concerned in the main with the findings in the Report on awareness, in thought and action, of the importance of nutrition at the national level. All figures shown in brackets in this part represent the percentage of the responding countries concerned as indicated by the Report. Part II makes some observations on the awareness in thought and action within the international community and at regional level. Part III comprises a number of general suggestions.

PART I: SOME CONCLUSIONS DRAWN FROM FINDINGS IN THE REPORT
AWARENESS IN THOUGHT AND ACTION AT THE NATIONAL LEVEL

The findings in the Report justify one broad conclusion. There is a growing awareness among governments of the importance of nutrition, first, in overall development, secondly, in early childhood, and thirdly, in the function of nutrition education to assist in building up the capacity to learn and to function. National nutritional goals and programmes, together with the necessary institutional arrangements for their formulation and implementation, stand a better chance than ever before of being established and of leading to nutrition education designed to assist in improving the total nutritional situation.

The phrase 'to assist' is introduced advisedly to draw attention to the limit there is to what the formal systems of education can be expected to do for the improvement of the nutritional situation. This is reflected in the findings of the Report regarding the levels at which nutrition education is introduced. Secondary education is mentioned by 83 per cent of responding countries followed by primary (75 per cent) and pre-school education (45 per cent). Seventy-eight per cent have incorporated the subject in their teacher-training programmes. Only 2 per cent have no plans for introducing nutrition studies at the secondary level, 5 per cent at the primary and 3 per cent at the teacher-training level. The picture is encouraging, if it is considered by itself without reference to the small proportion of populations that may be reached through school and college.

The figures tell a different story, however, when taken together with the high percentages of no response by countries in respect of populations in the maternity age-group of from 15 to 45 years (22 per cent) and the age-group of 50 to 60 years (48 per cent). The latter were so high 'most likely because these groups are not reached through the traditional educational systems'. It is also likely that many of these are neither reached by any other systems at all nor involved directly or indirectly in school activities that have to do with nutrition education. This may be inferred from a recent evaluation report on a Nutrition Project for 11- to 16-year-old pupils in Ghana, who ranked school, family, and religion, as institutions that influence them most. The evaluators conclude: 'Our experience showed that ideas in nutrition education can trickle through pupils from the school setting into the homes of the pupils. But a more efficient way of spreading information on the subject, however, is to involve parents directly in some school activities that have to do with nutrition education (Unesco Nutrition Education Project: Report by Curriculum Division, Ghana Education Service, Accra. July 1977, para. 5.2).

A greater involvement of the two age-groups and more attention to their own nutrition education are indicated to be necessary by the findings of the Report regarding public awareness of the importance of nutrition. Responding governments which were 'very aware' (52 per cent) themselves or 'partly aware' (35 per cent) assessed their public as being 'partly aware' (58 per cent) with a small number (5 per cent) vouching for a high level of awareness among the public. The figures for those who assessed parents (45 per cent) and the public (40 per cent) as 'partly aware' are rather high and raise the question as to whether quantitatively adequate feeding is not, in some cases, being substituted for good nutrition without a conscious awareness of the experience of the last two decades of the interrelations of quantity and quality of feeding (World Food Council: Report by the Executive Director WFC/41, 25 March 1977, para. 8). The view by responding countries of the North American sub-region that, 'while the public is aware of the importance of nutrition, it is not always aware of what constitutes good nutrition', is a fair conclusion and an argument for adequate attention to non-formal education in nutrition outside the school and college.

Another set of findings of the Report would seem to argue for a search for alternative but complementary systems of delivery to the formal educational systems. Perceivable awareness of the importance of nutrition on the one hand and of nutrition education on the other is reported to be in action, at least at two levels. First, responding countries (47 per cent) report that they have institutional arrangements for the establishment of food and nutrition policies and planning. Some countries (22 per cent) have not yet decided on arrangements and others (17 per cent) have approved schemes which have yet to be implemented. Arrangements in existence range from autonomous food or nutrition bodies, academic institutes, and programmes to units within ministries and departments of governments. Some responding countries (55 per cent) indicate that their national educational authorities are actively involved in the planning of nutritional policies. But others (37 per cent) record a relatively inactive involvement. Approximately the same proportions (53 per cent and 38 per cent) respectively indicate 'active' and 'relatively inactive' involvement of national educational authorities in the implementation of policies. Whatever the reasons for the relatively limited part which educational authorities consequently have in influencing thought and action in this important area of planning, they do not appear to be in the front line of attack on the problem of mal- and under-nutrition.

Secondly, 43 and 50 per cent of responding countries refer to

educators respectively as paying 'much attention' and 'some attention', in their work and concerns, to the widespread observation that
better nutrition is conducive to better learning. Forty-eight and 38
per cent respectively rate them as regarding their craft to be a 'very
important' and 'somewhat important' instrument in improving the
national nutritional level. The 10 per cent of countries whose educational practitioners consider the role of education as being 'not
very important' would seem to lend weight to the conclusion that
education is at present as limited in what it can do to bring about
change in food habits of its clients as in other areas of individual
and social living against a background where, as it is felt in the North
American region, 'the improvement of the nutritional situation is
not yet a conscious goal of educators'.

The African responses recorded as being of 'a wide variation in the
degree of emphasis . . . on education as an instrument for improving
nutrition' are noteworthy. 'Some placed no priority on education
while others felt that only in schools could one find a captive audience.' Twenty years ago the emphasis placed on education in school
and college as an instrument in improving the nutritional situation
would have been uniformly high among responding African governments. The discovery, since then, that formal systems have developed
more by good luck than by successful planning for a small élite and
that they are being called upon to perform functions for the masses
in rural Africa for which the systems had not been designed, has led
to a search for alternatives outside the school and college as well as
for a greater relevance within the systems themselves. That education
itself has to change and at the same time contribute to change is a
serious limiting factor regarding what it can do.

An appreciation of this fact would seem to underscore the North-
West European view in the Report that 'the existence of a national
nutrition policy would be more effective in improving nutrition and
that changes in economic status influenced eating habits at a much
faster rate than education'. If such a policy concerned itself more
with providing guidelines for maintaining harmonizing arrangements
for increasing the potential of all kinds of nutritional activities for
mutual reinforcement and less with setting out directives and achieving 'co-ordination', education in school and college would stand a
good chance, along with other social and cultural services functioning
outside them, of making its most effective contribution, in spite of
its own limitations.

The establishment of a national nutrition policy presupposes a
follow-up in the provision of the necessary facilities and personnel
for its implementation. The Report lists two categories of difficulties

that stand in the way of implementing nutrition education. One category comprises the familiar ones which have confronted the introduction into timetables of new subjects like African History into African schools in the 1950s and 1960s. Among these are lack of adequately prepared teachers in terms of subject-matter mentioned by 83 per cent of responding countries, teaching facilities (67 per cent), materials and equipment (68 per cent), time within the curricula (65 per cent), and adequate government support (40 per cent). Their solution rests mainly with decision-makers at the political and management levels, who are in a position to make funds available and stimulate the planning required to prepare educational personnel, to integrate the requisite nutritional learning experiences in curricula, and to provide the required administration and organization to support teaching.

The second category of difficulties is mentioned by much smaller numbers. These are unwillingness of teachers to make the change (30 per cent), public resistance to new or different subject-matter (25 per cent), and students' (children and adults) lack of interest (20 per cent). Although these difficulties are more serious because they have, more often than not, no rational basis and do not lend themselves to an easy solution, they are less common than the first type. They therefore augur well for nutrition education and seem to emphasize the need for more self-education at the level of decision-making until awareness is replaced by a deep concern; and there is incontrovertible evidence that much more than 52 per cent of their number are not only 'very aware' of the importance of nutrition in overall development and give unqualified support to nutrition education but also are convinced of the justice inscribed in the rubrics of the questionnaire: 'To attack illiteracy without simultaneously attacking mal- and undernutrition which hamper learning capacity seems hopeless, to put it mildly.'

PART II: OBSERVATIONS

AWARENESS IN THOUGHT AND ACTION–THE INTERNATIONAL LEVEL

When awareness adequately deepens into concern, the relevant need is highlighted within the councils and forums of the international community in general and of the appropriate specialized agency or agencies of the UN system in particular. The international community then comes up with the necessary budget to meet the cost of programmes and personnel to be involved. Something of the impressive scale in which the international community went into action, once awareness of decades of the handicap imposed by illiteracy had matured into a concern, may be seen in what it did in projects in Africa alone in the World Experimental Literacy Programme and subsequently in other areas, as shown in Table 17.1. In contrast, the international community has yet to give a similarly deserved emphasis to nutrition education and to match rhetoric with the reality of programme and budget. An examination of current provision discloses an appreciable measure of international concern about one need, which is yet to apply to the other in relation to which 'children may suffer irreversible mental and physical damage' (Report by the Executive Director, World Food Council, WFC/41, March 1977, para. 10).

And yet the cause of literacy would be immensely assisted if nutrition education were given the maximum chance at least of helping to protect the millions of one- to five-year-old children all over the world against the risk of xerophthalmia, and consequently incapacitate them for the literacy classes, to which so much import-ance is understandably attached. Indeed, one might go further. It would seem that good nutrition is a prerequisite for good literacy and numeracy, and since nobody argues against the thesis that 'no other curricular aims should deflect primary teachers from teaching literacy and numeracy', should not nutrition and health studies in the long term complete the trilogy? By definition, there is a case for the three forming part of the core of learning, the protected area of the curriculum in many parts of the less developed world, and remain so into the secondary level. If this was thought to be reason-able, then it should be of interest to the international community.

AWARENESS AT THE REGIONAL LEVEL

Awareness of any kind at the regional level is more difficult to assess than at the international. Available information shows, however, that evidence of regional interest in nutrition and health education, which was previously hard to come by in reports of regional meetings of Ministries of Education, National Commissions for UNESCO*, and of specialists in UNESCO's fields of competence, is beginning to appear at this level.

For example, the Conference of Ministers of Education of African Member States at Lagos in 1976 noted that the 'education in the theory and practice, health and nutrition education' currently taking place in some African countries is 'an aspect of the effort to make

*A National Commission for UNESCO is a National Group of representatives of govern-mental authorities as well as of national professional organizations, university institutes, and non-governmental organizations working in the fields of education, science, culture, and communication. It acts as the centre by which the national intellectual resources can be associated with the work of UNESCO, in the preparation, implementation, and evalu-ation of the Organization's programme.

Table 17.1

Functional literacy experimental projects in Africa (ED-76/MINEDAF/Ref. 5)
(All except that in Guinea were large-scale projects)

Country	Duration of international assistance	Population reached	Target envisaged in plan of operation	Cost, in dollars, per successful participant showing research cost in brackets	Areas of concentration including export crops and minor industries promoted
Algeria	1967–74	58 866	100 000	98 (15)	Management training; production of citrus fruits
Ethiopia	1968–73	38 000	100 000	92 (28)	Linguistic integration; coffee; textiles
Guinea	1968–71	1 440	78 000	208 (96)	Political integration; production of pineapple and rice; animal husbandry; carpentry; textiles; production of cigarettes, matches
Madagascar	1968–71	4 299	51 000	125 (48)	Rural development; production of rice, coffee, cotton; animal husbandry

Country	Duration of international assistance	Population reached	Target envisaged in plan of operation	Cost, in dollars, per successful participant showing research cost in brackets	Areas of concentration including export crops and minor industries promoted
Mali	1967–72	83 000	100 000	34 (20)	Civic responsibility; production of cotton, groundnuts, rice
Sudan	1969–73	7 385	16 000	271 (110)	Transition from nomadism to sedentary occupations; production of cotton, groundnuts, wheat; handicrafts; leather; oil; textiles
Tanzania	1967–73	466 000	200 000	10.46 (2)	Involvement in nation-building; animal husbandry; fishing; production of bananas, cotton, rice

At the peak of the programme in 1971–1972 UNESCO Member States approved a headquarters and field supporting staff of 1 Director and 35 professional and general service personnel and made available from the regular budget of their Organization and extra-budgetary sources $2.308 million and $4.681 million to meet the cost of staff and to provide the necessary intellectual support, equipment, and training facilities for nationals in all the four regions. The figures are insignificant; but taken together with the local operating costs and compared with the income per capita of the populations concerned, they represent a considerable outlay.

educational systems more relevant' (Final Report, 1976, para. 15). This represents a noteworthy advance following, as it did, the absence of any mention of nutrition and health education in the report of two preparatory missions which had preceded the Conference, assessed the interest of UNESCO African Member States in the establishment of a Network of Educational Innovations in Africa (NEIDA), and identified some of the problems and experiences on which Member States would like to exchange information (Report ED-76/MINEDAF/REF.3, 1 December 1975. Problems and experiences identified included Functional Literacy and Cooperation).

Developments in Asia have already brought NEIDA's predecessor, the Asian Programme of Educational Innovation for Development (APEID, established in January 1975), to a decision by its nineteen participating countries to include 'Better Health and Nutrition' among five 'common priority concerns' which innovations in education should contribute to and promote, the other four being Integrated Rural Development; Development of Productive Skills relevant to Economic Development; Universalization of Education for Out-of-School Youth and Adults; and National Unity and International Understanding and Cooperation (Final Report: Fourth Regional Consultation Meeting on APEID, Bangkok, April 1977, p. 46). The decision has been followed by the elaboration of work plans (see Annex I) setting out the implications of the decision in objectives and expected outcomes for seven areas of innovation: Non-formal and alternative structures in education; administration and management; curriculum development; educational technology; preparation of teachers, teacher educators, and other educational personnel; science (including mathematics) and technology education; and vocational education (Work Plans of APEID for 1978-1981, Bangkok, 1977, pp. 71-4.)

The support which APEID has decided to give to education for better nutrition and health is likely to go far for several reasons. The programme is determined and approved by national authorities themselves, and priority areas are defined at the regional level by matching needs expressed and resources offered. It encourages the utilization of existing national expertise and capacity for development wherever they may be found—within and outside higher educational institutions. It has an in-built system of evaluation, and the opportunity of learning by decision-makers from the successes and failures of one another is available. With more self-financing with a view to becoming self-supporting, it promises to be an economical mechanism for internal assistance to Member States. It obviates the need for conscious planning and establishment of centres of excellence but encourages growth towards excellence as experience is built up for carrying out the work dictated by identified common priority concerns.

If education for better nutrition and health secured a similar place in the four counterparts of APEID now at different stages of evolution—NEIDA in Africa, the Educational Innovation Programme for Development in Arab States (EIPDAS), the Carribean and South-East European networks—awareness of the importance of nutrition education would stand a better chance of being developed. That may, in turn, hopefully lead to a stronger voice on its behalf within the international community and at other regional meetings like those of Ministries of Education and National Commissions for UNESCO and thereby win deserving support for effort at the national level.

PART III: SUGGESTIONS

A major suggestion that can be made at this stage is that the APEID development should be studied, and similar regional efforts should be encouraged.

The four counterparts of APEID—NEIDA in Africa, EIPDAS in the Arab States, and the Caribbean and south-east European networks—should, at the appropriate points in their development, be invited to give consideration in their programmes to the following observations: (i) 'how much an individual (adult or child) can take advantage of educational opportunities offered depends to a large extent on his or her physical and mental fitness and well-being'; (ii) 'proper nutrition contributes greatly to physical and mental health'; and (iii) improvement of nutrition and health involves, among other things, 'awareness and understanding of basic knowledge pertaining to health, hygiene, and nutrition; and development of proper attitudes towards health, hygiene, environment, nutrition, and the formation of good health and food habits'.

Regional co-operative endeavours promoting education in nutrition and health would need, first, to be flexible in their arrangements, to enable them to reflect changing needs of the participating countries and, second, to earn and benefit from the support of regional or sub-regional organizations already involved in this field—REIDA from OAU, EIPDAS from the Arab Educational, Cultural and Scientific Organization (ALECSO); the Caribbean network from the Caribbean Development and Co-operation Committee (CDCC), and the South-East European network from sub-regional and bilateral arrangements.

Governmental and non-governmental organizations interested in nutrition and health education as a priority concern should examine the prospects of such regional co-operative exchange mechanisms to find out in which ways they can be used as: a source of necessary self-education of decision-makers, a point of entry for their own members as individual specialists or affiliated groups of specialists to contribute expertise, and, a means of promoting the cause of nutrition and health education.

Nutrition and health education should be recognized as only one basic source which should complement, reinforce, and be reinforced by other basic sources that provide and make available basic/primary medical and health care, ensure capacity to obtain proper food, and health amenities, including adequate housing and social welfare, train the necessary paramedical and extension agricultural workers (including voluntary social and health workers); and safeguard the environment within which health and nutrition education has to be practised.

The limit that there is to what school and college can achieve in many countries is in itself a strong recommendation for making non-formal and alternative structures in education a priority area of innovation for facilitating activities in out-of-school nutrition and health education, focusing on local initiative and participation, full use of local resources, and the development of the community for the purpose of raising nutrition and health standards.

Maintaining activities in school and out-of-school as complementary and mutually reinforcing efforts would require the support of pedagogical higher educational institutions in the search for: (i) the kind of learning experiences which should be incorporated in curricula and at what stages; (ii) the best way the requisite learning can be encouraged and practised; (iii) the best means of assessing the efficiency of selected learning experiences in terms of what they achieve and of finding out how the beneficiaries perform as individuals and as members of society; and (iv) the best type of training required by trained personnel to use the organization available effectively and guide the learning, practice, and evaluation necessary. These are predominantly pedagogical functions.

The search for suitable learning experiences should take into consideration, where applicable, the place of the selection, preparation, and sharing of food in indigenous education as an educative process together with the value system of which they are a part. This calls for a careful examination of, and selection from, the different designs in existence for curriculum-construction, for example, a design:

(1) whereby activities are chosen because they can be assumed to produce certain behaviours desired from students after a period of instruction; or

(2) which calls for greater participation on the part of students in the curriculum-making process, placing some faith upon the contacts the students make with what is provided in school, home, and community in general and parents in particular; or

(3) which makes the student the central factor and gives him the opportunity to decide what he wants to know and when he wants to learn it; or

(4) a combination of some or all as appropriate.

The preparation of personnel for the tasks of nutrition education, of which the continuing self-education of decision-makers that can take place within the framework of networks of educational innovations for development must form a part, constitutes the key to the solution of problems in that field. The category, however, which requires so much attention is that of the practitioner who requires not only to know nutrition in terms of subject-matter but to have insights which come from scientific training in the art of education, which help him to understand students, appreciate how they learn and what changes can reasonably be expected in their behaviour, attitudes, and habits after a period of instruction.

An impressive list of countries from which nutrition educators from 29 states have had their training is provided in Table 35 of the Report and is included here as Annex II. There is the need to ensure, as one of the tasks of the future, that training at all levels of personnel at home or in foreign countries provides both the substance of nutrition and the science of education. There is also the need to build up an information and advisory service on where the combined training is obtainable.

A necessary parallel step would be to ensure that regional co-operative endeavours which make nutrition education a common priority concern contribute to, and benefit from, such a service through association with centres of training that fulfil the criteria of provision of specialized nutrition and education training.

Finally, the harmonizing arrangements required at the national level to hold together in a mutually helpful relationship the activities in nutrition education in and out of school, of other basic services, and of the training of personnel are of paramount importance. The national education authorities can play a significant part in the formulation of these from a position of understanding of the relationship between good nutrition and good education and of a commitment to the cause of Better Nutrition and Better Education.

REFERENCE

Gordon, H.F. and Calloway D.H. (1977). *Position of Nutrition Education within Educational Systems*, UNESCO, Paris.

Annex I

Work plans of APEID for 1978–1981

Development Theme: Better Health and Nutrition

1. *Area of Innovation: Non-formal and Alternative Structures in Education*
   Objectives:
   1. To facilitate innovations in education focusing on local initiative, partici-
      pation, full use of local resources and development of the community in
      raising health and nutrition standards; and
   2. To facilitate inter-agency co-operation in identifying educational needs
      and programmes for better health and nutrition.

   Expected outcomes:
   A. Increased co-operation amongst the existing agencies concerned with
      health and nutrition in order to promote, through education, changes in
      attitudes, values and habits; and
   B. Increased sharing of experiences and collaboration amongst Member
      States in the use of non-formal and new structures in education to raise
      levels of health and nutrition.

2. *Area of Innovation: Administration and Management of Educational
   Innovations*
   Objectives:
   1. To facilitate development of information on health and nutrition to
      develop more effective supervisory systems and practices for raising the
      standards of health and nutrition of pupils and community awareness of
      such problems; and
   2. To promote co-ordination of inter-departmental efforts in the field of
      health and nutrition, so that the reorganized systems and knowledge
      gained can be used for education.

   Expected outcomes:
   A. Increased collaboration in sharing experiences and basic data on health
      and nutrition in the community; and
   B. Greater involvement of the community in relating education to better
      health and nutrition.

3. *Area of Innovation: Curriculum Development*
   Objectives:
   1. To strengthen the capacities for developing relevant approaches and
      methodologies of curriculum preparation and relevant instructional
      materials, utilizing local resources with emphasis on promoting awareness
      and basic understanding of principles underlying the theme and integration
      of the basic concepts relevant to the theme in different disciplines; and
   2. To facilitate the development of flexible institutional structures and
      procedures.

   Expected outcomes:
   A. Data on alternative structures in curriculum development (including
      radio/TV programmes) for better health, hygiene, nutrition and balanced
      diet; and

B. Training of concerned personnel and other voluntary organizations for designing and developing curricula and teaching material, in relation to the community's needs for health, hygiene and nutrition.

4. *Area of Innovation: Educational Technology*

Objectives:

1. To use indigenous games, dance, music, drama and other modes, as well as available mass media for promoting proper health and nutrition concepts and habits; and
2. To develop teaching aids and self-instructional packages relevant to health, hygiene and nutrition.

Expected outcome:

A. Fuller participation of the people in developing awareness for the improvement of health, hygiene and nutrition habits.

5. *Area of Innovation: Education of Teachers, Teacher Educators and Other Educational Personnel*

Objectives:

1. To enhance national capacities for developing relevant approaches and methodologies for teacher education and training programmes for education in better health, nutrition and family welfare in the community; and
2. To promote development of teaching materials involving interdisciplinary and multi-media approaches and the use of community resources for education in better health, nutrition and family welfare in the community.

Expected outcomes:

A. Development of better understanding and insight into the interdisciplinary nature of training educational personnel for health and nutrition education.
B. Relevant data and information obtained from analysing innovative experiences in preparing teachers and other educational personnel for health and nutrition education.

6. *Area of Innovation: Science (including Mathematics) and Technology Education*

Objectives:

Through support to national initiative and regional exchange of experiences and their synthesis, develop national capabilities:

1. to identify key concepts and processes of science and to develop practical activities leading to the provision of more effective learning experiences in order to develop positive attitudes toward health, nutrition, hygiene, sanitation and environmental awareness; and
2. to survey existing practices and innovative measures in Member States leading to a more relevant and improved formal and non-formal education in these fields.

Expected outcomes:

A. Improved community practices in health, nutrition, sanitation and hygiene;
B. Greater sensitivity to environmental problems; and
C. Data on community practices on production, preservation and preparation of foods.

7. *Area of Innovation: Vocational Education*

Objectives:

Through exchange of experiences and co-operative efforts, enhance national capabilities:

1. to develop appropriate vocational education courses and instructional materials to provide a sound base for training of technicians in the fields of health, sanitation, nutrition and family welfare, both in formal and non-formal education; and
2. to develop effective learning-teaching experiences related to health, nutrition, diet management, food preservation and preparation, animal husbandry and fishery.

Expected outcomes:

A. Enhancement of knowledge and techniques of vocational education curriculum design and construction, to meet the needs of programmes for better health and nutrition; and
B. Better community awareness, understanding and habits with respect to health and nutrition.

Annex II

Training of nutrition educators in other than native country

Native country	Country in which training took place	Educational level reached	Level(s) taught
Africa			
Congo	France	University	Secondary
Ghana	United Kingdom	B.Sc.,Ph.D.	University, secondary
	USA	B.Sc., M.PH.	University, secondary
	Canada	B.A.	Teacher training
	West Germany	Ph.D.	University
Ivory Coast	France	Graduate, post-graduate	All levels
	Germany	Graduate, and post-graduate	All levels
	Italy	Graduate	All levels
	Canada	Graduate and post-graduate	All levels
	Belgium	Graduate and post-graduate	All levels
Kenya	United Kingdom	Post-graduate	University
	USA	Undergraduate	University, and teacher-training
	Nigeria	Post-graduate	Ministry of Health
	Israel	Diploma course	Ministry of Health
Liberia	USA	University	Community schools
	European countries	Short courses	Training programmes Adult education Home economics University community development

Native country	Country in which training took place	Educational level reached	Level(s) taught
Africa (contd.)			
Nigeria	United Kingdom	University	Secondary
	USA	Post-graduate	University
	Australia	Doctorate	University
	Canada		
	Israel		
Senegal	France	ENNA	Normal schools
Somalia	India	University	Secondary, teacher-training
Upper Volta	France	University	Secondary
	Israel	University	Secondary
	Belgium	University	Secondary
Zambia	USA	University	Post-secondary
	United Kingdom	University	Secondary
	Australia	Secondary	Teacher-training
Arab States			
Egypt	United Kingdom	B.Sc. and Ph.D.	
	USA	B.Sc. and Ph.D.	
Iraq	United Kingdom	M.Sc. and Ph.D.	High school,
	USA	M.Sc. and Ph.D.	university
Jordan	Egypt	M.Sc. and B.Sc. Foods and Nutrition	Teacher-training
Asia, South West			
India	USA	Post-doctorate	University
Iran	USA	Teacher	University
	United Kingdom	Ph.D., M.Ph.	Institutes
	France	D.S.	
	Germany		
Sri Lanka	United Kingdom	Post-graduate	Undergraduate, post-graduate
	USA		
	India		
Asia, South East			
Indonesia	USA	Certificate	Undergraduate,
	Canada	Masters Degree	graduate
	India		
	United Kingdom		
Malaysia	United Kingdom	B.Ed.	Teacher-training
	Australia	Diploma & Specialist	Primary, secondary
	Indonesia	Home Science Certificate Diploma, Applied Nutrition	Vocational
Phillipines	USA	Post-graduate	High school, under-graduate and graduate
	England	Post-graduate	
	Canada		

Native country	Country in which training took place	Educational level reached	Level(s) taught
Asia, South East (contd.)			
	Australia	Post-graduate	High-school, under-graduate and graduate
	India		
	Japan		Elementary, high school, graduate and post-graduate
	Holland		
	Belgium	Post-graduate	
	Thailand		
	Israel		Elementary, high school, graduate and post-graduate
Singapore	New Zealand	University	Nursing school,
	United Kingdom	University	Teacher-training
	USA	University	Graduate, post-graduate
	Australia	University	Teacher-training
Thailand	USA	University	University, college, and high school
	Europe		
	Philippines	University	
	India		
	New Zealand		
Asia, Far East			
Korea	USA	Doctorate	Undergraduate,
	W. Germany	Masters Diploma	graduate
	Japan	Certificate	Junior College
	France		Teacher-training
	England		
	Canada		
	Australia		
Oceania			
Australia	United Kingdom	M.S.	Secondary
	USA	Ph.D.	Tertiary
	Canada		
	New Zealand		
	India		
New Zealand	United Kingdom	Ph.D.	University
	USA	Post Doctoral	University
Europe, Northern/Western			
Ireland	United Kingdom	Nutrition Courses	University
	USA		
Netherlands	United Kingdom	M.Sc. Ph.D.	University
	USA		
Sweden	USA	University	Teacher-training
	Norway	Masters Degree	Secondary

Native country	Country in which training took place	Educational level reached	Level(s) taught
Europe, Northern/Western (contd.)			
United Kingdom	USA Canada	University	Secondary University
Europe, Southern			
Cyprus	Greece United Kingdom USA	University	Primary, secondary, adult education
Latin America			
Argentina	USA France Panama	University	Secondary, university
Barbados	Canada USA United Kingdom	University	Secondary, and tertiary
Colombia	Mexico USA Puerto Rico Guatemala Brazil	University, post-university	University
Costa Rica	Argentina Guatemala Mexico	University	Secondary Technical University
Guatemala	USA Puerto Rico Belgium	Undergraduate Graduate	Undergraduate Graduate
Guyana	USA Jamaica United Kingdom	B.Sc., M.Sc., Diploma	Teacher-training High School University
Montserrat	Jamaica Puerto Rico		Junior secondary Secondary
Panama	Argentina Guatemala Colombia USA Mexico	Licensed nutritionists and dieticians	III & IV graduate

18 A review of the activities of the FAO in nutrition education and training 1949-1977

JEAN W. McNAUGHTON

INTRODUCTION

The World Food Conference in Rome in 1974 focused the attention of the world community on the fact that millions of people were hungry and malnourished in spite of the brave words about 'freedom from want' that were part of the Declaration of Human Rights. Not since the end of the Second World War in 1945, when blueprints for the various United Nations Agencies were being drawn up, has there been so much discussion about the need for policies and programmes to improve nutrition. Both explicitly and implicitly there has been the recognition that actions taken since the Second World War by the various bodies with a mandate to improve nutrition have not brought about the hoped-for results. Criticism has been directed at international agencies and at governments. The mood is to wipe the slate clean, to turn one's back on the past, and begin again. This approach appeals to the child and the optimist in most of us. I have long felt that Stewart Chase's salutary *The Proper Study of Mankind*, which shows that we seldom learn from the past, should be compulsory reading for anyone involved in decision-making or programme-planning.

Before we consider what the FAO should or can do in the future to assist governments to strengthen nutrition education and training it might be instructive to review briefly what the FAO has done in the past and to attempt to assess the successes and failures, and to see what lessons we can learn from these.

I wish to make it clear that many of the FAO activities in nutrition education and training, as is the case for our other nutrition activities, are joint endeavours with our sister organizations of the UN family, the WHO, UNESCO, and UNICEF. We also collaborate and co-operate with other inter-governmental bodies. For example, for a number of years the FAO had joint nutrition education and training programmes with the South Pacific Commission, the now defunct Caribbean Commission, and more recently with the Women's Training and Research Centre of the Economic Commission for Africa. The FAO's participation in the Centre is effected through the secondment of two staff members, both nutrition educators, of the Planning

for Better Family Living Unit, Home Economics and Social Programmes Service. Perhaps, too, I should point out that the FAO's
nutrition education and training assistance to member governments
may be channelled through the Food Policy and Nutrition Division
or the Home Economics and Social Programmes Service of the
Human Resources, Institutions, and Agrarian Reform Division. The
Food Policy and Nutrition Division and the Home Economics
and Social Programmes Service work closely together in developing
the nutrition content of home economics programmes and in nutrition training in agriculture.

AN OVERVIEW OF THE FAO's NUTRITION EDUCATION AND
TRAINING ACTIVITIES 1949–1977

The nutrition education and training activities can be grouped under
the following headings:

(a) assessment of training needs;
(b) technical assistance in strengthening nutrition education and training; and
(c) preparation of training materials.

Assessment of training needs

From the beginning the UN agencies concerned with nutrition decided
that lack of trained personnel was a major constraint to improving
nutrition. The Report of the Second Session of the Joint FAO/WHO
Expert Committee on Nutrition (1951) states 'In many under-
developed countries there is a lack of personnel trained in nutrition
who can contribute to the improvement of the nutritional status of
the population. In such circumstances the training of the necessary
personnel of different kinds is of primary importance.' The report
goes on to list the various kinds of personnel who need training, and
the type of training needed. Four categories of personnel were
identified: (a) professional nutritionists to staff a central nutrition
service, (b) staff at central level in ministries of agriculture, health,
education, etc. with responsibility for planning and organizing
nutrition programmes within their own ministries, (c) district or
local staff of these agencies with responsibility for improving nutrition, i.e. public-health and medical officers, public-health nurses,
community-development workers, agriculture and home-economics
extension workers and teachers, and (d) village-level field staff,
local officials, and village leaders.

The Joint FAO-WHO Expert Committee continued to be very
concerned about the need for nutrition education and training. The
Report of the Fourth Committee (1955) contains an Annex setting
out methods and content of education in nutrition. The Fifth

Committee held in 1957, the Sixth Committee in 1961, and the Eighth Committee in 1970 reiterated the need for trained personnel and assessed achievements briefly. The Ninth Committee in 1974 considered training needs in relation to the planning and implemen= tation of food and nutrition policy and pointed out that knowledge about food and nutrition problems and possible solutions must reach two extreme points, on the one side the top government decision-makers and on the other the needy population who are predominantly the rural poor. The Committee defined six categories of personnel to be trained. It is interesting to note that its categories are essentially the same as those of the Second Joint Committee, but it splits the fourth group into three, namely local government administrators and field staff of technical agencies (health, agriculture, education, etc.) concerned with co-ordination of government services at local level, key personnel in each community (political, social, and religious leaders, etc.), and local auxilliary workers. The Committee decided there was no global answer to training, each country must assess its own personnel requirements and decide how to allocate its resources for training. It did, however, suggest that priority should be given to training the staff needed to provide food and nutrition services at the community level and identified the need for training multi-purpose workers, for training their trainers and for inter-sectoral training.

In addition to the discussions on training by the Joint FAO–WHO Committee, the FAO, either alone or jointly with the WHO, has organized a number of regional and national meetings on nutrition education and training, and has made several assessments of training needs. One example of historic interest is the Survey of Nutrition Education in six Western European countries (France, Belgium, the Netherlands, Federal Republic of Germany, Italy, and the United Kingdom) made by a FAO–WHO mission in 1961. It would be interesting to repeat that survey, and record the progress made in the interval in these countries, as well as discussing the problems that were encountered in strengthening university-level training in nutrition.

Several years ago we attempted an inventory of personnel with professional training in nutrition in Africa south of the Sahara and in Latin America, as a basis for projections of training needs for these regions. If my memory is correct, at that time there were between 90 and 100 nutritionists employed in Africa, more than half of them expatriates, while there were more than 400 profession-ally trained nutritionists in Latin America.

More recently (1975–7) an assessment of facilities for training in nutrition and food science research in countries in Africa south of the Sahara was carried out by three consultants for the FAO Regional Office for Africa.

Technical assistance in strengthening nutrition education and training

These activities are being carried out by staff members from Headquarters or the Regional Offices under the Regular Programme and by consultants funded under the United Nations Development Programme, UNICEF, the FAO–Government Co-operative Programme or other trust funds.

Assistance has been provided for training at professional level for personnel to head training units in universities, colleges, and other institutions, for research workers to staff nutrition institutes, for extension workers in applied nutrition programmes, home economics, and nutrition services, and for local field-workers in nutrition programmes. Training at university level and in other institutions of higher learning has usually been through the provision of fellowships for training abroad and through consultants to help set up institutions in member countries. For extension workers it has been either through fellowships abroad or through institutions of higher learning and through specialized short in-service training. Local field-workers have been trained largely through in-service training programmes. Training materials and equipment have also been provided.

Assistance was given to more than 60 countries in the decade 1961-70. Currently the Food Policy and Nutrition Division is involved with training activities in 18 countries.

In addition to assistance to individual countries, technical assistance in training has also been provided at the regional level. One of the first regional training programmes in nutrition began in 1961 as the 'Joint FAO/UNICEF Africa Training Programme in Nutrition and in Extension as related to Nutrition'. A series of four regional and ten national courses were held in French and English and more than 40 fellowships were granted to selected trainees. From 1963 to 1967 the School of Hygiene and Tropical Medicine, University of London and the University of Ibadan, Nigeria, assisted by the FAO, UNICEF and the WHO offered an international post-graduate inter-disciplinary certificate course in food science and applied nutrition. During that time 120 fellows, including 41 from eleven African countries, completed the course. Responsibility for the Course has now been taken over by the University of Ibadan with continued financial support from UNICEF. Two similar regional-level professional training courses for francophone Africans were organized in 1964 and 1966 in Paris, Dakar, and Tunis, and attended by 46 participants.

Between 1965 and 1973 a series of medium-level training courses in food and nutrition for African personnel working in agriculture and home-economics extension, community development, education, and health were offered by the Government of Israel with FAO and WHO sponsorship. UNICEF and UNESCO also provided fellowships.

In Latin America inter-disciplinary professional-level regional training courses designed primarily for graduates in agriculture were organized at La Molina University, Peru, and subsequently at Bogota National University, Colombia, with financial assistance from UNICEF and technical assistance from the FAO.

Beginning in 1970 a joint FAO–WHO–UNESCO–UNICEF Nutrition Training Project for the Near East funded largely by UNICEF has organized regional and national training courses, workshops, and seminars in the region. The FAO has also organized a series of regional training courses on nutrition and on home economics for medium-level workers in the Caribbean, and similar courses jointly with the WHO and UNICEF in the South Pacific.

Current regional training activities centre on seminars or workshops, on national food and nutrition planning, and on the organization and management of group feeding programmes, particularly those utilizing food-aid donated by the World Food Programme. Follow-up of the regional training through national training projects has already begun and will continue in the 1978–9 biennium.

By the late 1960s there was an increasing awareness that agriculturists, nutritionists, and food economists needed to collaborate closely in formulating programmes and policies to eradicate hunger. One of the factors hampering such collaboration was the absence in agricultural training programmes of a component covering the broad principle of human nutrition and food economics. The FAO has assisted a number of agricultural institutions with the introduction of human nutrition into their curricula (e.g. in Morocco, Ghana, Uganda, Liberia, Swaziland, India, Malaysia, and Tanzania) but human nutrition, food science, and food economics are still not included in the training of agriculture students in many developing countries.

Preparation of training materials

The FAO has been involved in the preparation of a large number of publications and of other training materials such as posters and filmstrips. These include publications and filmstrips for general use issued in English, Spanish, and French, and publications and other training materials prepared for use in a specific region or an individual country. In general publications for general use are funded by the FAO regular budget, while materials for specific training courses or for individual countries are prepared as part of a project and funded through it, either by UNDP or trust funds. The FAO Freedom from Hunger—Action for Development has funded a number of publications for use in nutrition education programmes at country level.

One of the earliest training materials was *Teaching better nutrition* by Jean Ritchie, which was issued in 1950 as FAO Nutritional Studies No. 6. Its revised edition, *Learning better nutrition* FAO Nutritional Studies came out in 1967 and continues to be a bestseller. Altogether 28 publications have been issued in the Nutritional Studies Series.

Another publication used widely is Latham's (1965) *Human nutrition in tropical Africa* published under the auspices of the FAO, WHO, and UNICEF which is now in its fifth printing. A revised edition, funded by Sweden through a trust fund with the FAO, is in preparation. The first edition of *Human nutrition in tropical Africa* was one of a series in a project to provide textbooks for Africa, funded by UNICEF.

A list of some of the FAO publications that have been widely used as training materials in member countries is included in the bibliography at the end of this chapter. Material prepared by FAO personnel in co-operation with their national counterparts in nutritional education and training projects in individual countries has not been included in the bibliography because of space limitations.

ASSESSMENT OF THE EFFECTIVENESS OF THE FAO's ACTIVITIES
IN NUTRITION EDUCATION AND TRAINING

I would like to insert an aside at this point. Currently there seem to be two sets of opinions in vogue with regard to the value of nutrition education and training. On the one hand there is a group which appears to believe that since malnutrition still exists nutrition education and training have achieved nothing and should be abandoned. On the other hand, many people support nutrition education activities uncritically in the belief that it is enough to teach people what to eat in order to improve nutrition. Both groups ignore the complex network of factors that influence food patterns and food consumption. Ecology and economic, cultural, and social factors all play a part in determining what we eat. Their relative importance varies within and between communities, and even for the same individual over time.

At the outset I must admit that there has been very little formal evaluation of the FAO's technical assistance in nutrition education and training. In spite of attention given to the methodology of evaluation from the middle 1960s on, and the organization jointly by the FAO and the WHO of technical meetings and regional seminars to provide orientation with regard to putting this methodology into practice, few projects collected systematically even simple data that would have served for evaluation. However, assessment of some projects has been carried out. In addition, project reports and other documentation enable some conclusions to be drawn about the positive and negative features of the nutrition education and training programmes which the FAO has assisted.

Nutrition institutes

In the 1950s and 1960s the FAO together with the WHO provided assistance for the establishment or strengthening of a number of nutrition institutes, including the two regional institutes, Institute for Nutrition for Central America and Panama (INCAP) and the Caribbean Food and Nutrition Institute (CFNI), which now have established reputations. Both institutions are still assisted by PAHO-WHO, but not by the FAO.

Unfortunately our budgetary limitations have precluded this. Experience with the regional institutes demonstrates that it is difficult for such institutions to be supported solely from within the region. The picture presented by the national institutions which received international assistance varies. Some are very active in helping establish policies and programmes to improve nutrition in their countries, others are doing competent research and some training but are not really a force in improving nutrition since the research undertaken has little relation to the needs of their countries. Unfortunately some national institutions are doing very little. Reasons for these differences include shortage of well-trained staff, lack of equipment and resources, the political structure of the countries, and the personality and training of the staff. One can identify here one weakness of international assistance, namely the failure to follow up fellows on their return from training abroad.

Training of nutrition workers

The results of fellowship training have been mixed, but on the whole positive, in spite of the problems familiar to many of us of finding institutions in developed countries which provide training at the undergraduate level suited to fellows who will return to a developing country. One negative aspect was mentioned above— failure to adapt the training received to the needs of their home countries. Another has been the wastage of fellows. Sometimes they do not return home at all, or on their return are assigned by their governments to posts which do not require the training they have received. In some cases, in spite of obligations, the fellow chooses other employment or is not employed by his government because of changes in government priorities.

Training of field-level nutrition workers is probably the weakest link in the chain of training activities, in spite of the large number and variety of training courses that have been organized for these personnel with FAO, WHO, and UNICEF assistance. Experience has shown that training for this group has often tended to be too theoretical, that trainees have not a clear understanding of nutrition information, that in addition they have not received sufficient instruction in what to teach and how to teach, nor, once trained, have they received supervision and guidance. Added to this, their numbers have often been small, so that the coverage achieved by the programme in which they are extension workers (agriculture, health, rural development) has been very small in relation to the need.

Although the FAO has organized many regional seminars and workshops for both professional and technician-level training our experience is that while these may provide opportunities for an exchange of experience, or for increasing the knowledge of individual participants, they have not as a whole made a large contribution to strengthening national institutions or training capacity. In part this has been due to participation by the wrong people, but to a much greater extent to the fact that one person with specialized training can make little impact. In view of this, the FAO is now concentrating more on national-level training than on regional training courses.

The other problem is how to make more impact at 'grass-root' level. Even with the accent that has been given to training extension workers, nutrition services are not reaching the majority of families in the developing countries and these are after all the ultimate targets of nutrition education.

THE FAO's FUTURE PLANS FOR NUTRITION EDUCATION AND TRAINING

In one sentence, these are to give top priority to strengthening programmes to improve the nutrition of the needy, particularly the rural poor. Our previous experience has taught us that this group is the most difficult to reach, but it is clear that unless they are reached the world community will not achieve the goals set for it in regard to improving nutrition with the present decade.

The training endeavours of the Food Policy and Nutrition Division are concentrated on the following areas:

(1) assisting governments to strengthen their capabilities in food and nutrition planning and surveillance;
(2) assisting, together with other Divisions of FAO, in the integration of nutritional objectives into food and agriculture development plans and in projects related to food production and supply, distribution, and consumption; and
(3) assisting with 'training the trainers' of grass-root-level workers in nutrition and supplementary feeding programmes.

REFERENCES

Ackroyd, W.R. and Doughty, J. (1964). *Legumes in human nutrition*. FAO Nutritional Studies No. 19.
— (1970). *Wheat in human nutrition*. FAO Nutritional Studies No. 23.
Chase, Stuart, and Brunner, E. de S. (1978). *The Proper Study of Mankind*. Greenwood Press, London.
Dema, I.S. (1965). *Nutrition in relation to agricultural production*.
— (1968). *Food composition tables for use in Africa*.
FAO (1973). *Resource lessons for domestic science in village polytechnics*.
— (1978). *Food, nutrition and agriculture. Guidelines for curriculum content in agricultural training*.
— (1979). Field programme management. *Food and nutrition: a training pack*.
— (1979). *Group feeding programme management: a training pack*. (In preparation.)
Holmes, A.C. (1968). *Visual aids in nutrition education*.
Home Economics and Social Programmes Service (1976). *Rural home techniques*: Vol. 1 *Food preservation*, Vol. 3 *Food preparation*.
Jardin, C. and Crosnier, J. (1975). *A taro, a fish, a papaya*. Manual for nutrition education and applied nutrition for teachers in tropical oceania. [Original title and manual in French.]
Johnston, B.F. and Greaves, J.P. (1969). *Manual on food and nutrition policy*. Nutritional Studies No. 22.
Joy, L. and Payne, P. (1975). *Food and nutrition planning*. FAO Nutrition Consultants' Reports Series No. 35.
Kon, S.K. (1972). *Milk and milk products in human nutrition*. FAO Nutritional Studies No. 27. (2nd revised edn.)
Latham, M.C. (1965). *Human nutrition in tropical Africa*.
Passmore, R. (1970). *Amino-acid content of foods*. FAO Nutrition Studies No. 24.
— (1973). Energy and protein requirements. FAO Nutrition Meetings Report Series No. 52.
— (1974). *Handbook on human nutritional requirements*. FAO Nutritional Studies No. 28.
Prosper, M.S. (1976). *Manual for school feeding*. [In French and Arabic.]
Richie,J.A.S. (1967). *Learning better nutrition*. FAO Nutritional Studies No. 20.
— (1971). *Food and nutrition education in the primary school*. FAO Nutritional Studies No. 25.

JOINT FAO–WHO EXPERT COMMITTEE REPORTS WHICH CONTAIN
RECOMMENDATIONS CONCERNING NUTRITION EDUCATION AND
TRAINING

FAO (1951). *Joint FAO/WHO Expert Committee on Nutrition. Report on the Second Session.* FAO Nutrition Meetings Report Series No. 5. Rome.

— (1955). *Joint FAO/WHO Expert Committee on Nutrition. Report of the Fourth Session.* FAO Nutrition Meetings Report Series No. 9. Rome.

— (1958). *Joint FAO/WHO Expert Committee on Nutrition. Fifth Report.* FAO Nutrition Meetings Report Series No. 19. Rome.

— (1962). *Joint FAO/WHO Expert Committee on Nutrition. Sixth Report.* FAO Nutrition Meetings Report Series No. 32. Rome.

— (1966). *Joint FAO/WHO Expert Committee on Nutrition. Seventh Report.* FAO Nutrition Meetings Report Series No. 42. Rome.

— (1971). *Joint FAO/WHO Expert Committee on Nutrition. Eighth Report.* FAO Nutrition Meetings Report Series No. 49. Rome.

— (1976). *Food and Nutrition Strategies in National Development. Ninth Report of the Joint FAO/WHO Expert Committee on Nutrition.* FAO Nutrition Meetings Report Series No. 56. Rome.

Selected FAO reports dealing with nutrition education and training

Berger, S. (1975). *Third report on higher education and training in food and nutrition at agricultural universities and colleges in India.*

Cheftel, C., (1976). *Formation et Recherches en nutrition et en science et technologie alimentaire au Cameroun, en Côte d'Ivoire et au Sénégal—rapport de mission.* [mimeo].

— (1976). *Formation et recherches en nutrition et en science et technologie alimentaire au Bénin, en Guinée, au Togo et au Zaire—rapport de Mission.* [mimeo].

FAO (1960). *Report of the Symposium on Education and Training in Nutrition in Europe, 1959.* FAO Nutrition Meetings Report Series No. 26.

— (1962). *Nutrition education in six Western European countries.* Report of an FAO/WHO mission.

— (1974). *Suggestions for courses in Home Technology, University Pertanian, Malaysia.*

— (1975). *Enseignement de la nutrition humaine et de l'economie alimentaire à L'Institut Agromique et Vétérinaire Hassan II, Maroc.* [French only].

— (1976). *The establishment of a three-year diploma course for women in agriculture and home economics, Egerton College, Kenya.*

— (1975, 1976, 1977). Series: rapports pour les Républiques populaires du Bénin et du Congo, l'Empire centrafricain, le Gabon, la Rwanda, la Haute-Volta, le Cameroun. [French only].

Truswell, S. (1976). *Consultancy report: review and recommendations on nutrition food science and technology, training and research activities in Ghana, Kenya, Sierra Leone, Sudan and Tanzania.* [mimeo].

Selected publications on planning and evaluation of nutrition programmes including education and training

Garine, I. de (1964). *Planificacion y evalución de programas de nutrición aplicade en América Latina (Chile, Paraguay y Brazil).*

McArthur, M. (1964). *Study for the improvement of applied nutrition projects planning in Africa.*
— (1965). *Report of the joint FAO/WHO technical meeting on methods of planning and evaluation in applied nutrition programmes.* FAO Nutrition Meetings Report Series No. 39.
Latham, M.C. (1972). *Planning and evaluation of applied nutrition programmes.* FAO Nutritional Studies No. 26.

19 UNICEF co-operation in educational efforts to improve nutrition

BRIGITTE TRIMMER-SMITH AND L.J. TEPLEY

THE EARLY YEARS

The United Nations International Children's Emergency Fund (UNICEF) was established in 1946. Its primary aim for the first few years of its existence was to provide emergency supplies in the form of food, clothing, medicine, school books, etc., for mothers and young children suffering the aftermath of the Second World War and natural disasters. In Europe, for instance, approximately 6 million children received a daily supplementary meal through 50 000 centres in twelve countries, and distribution of milk-powder was a major activity. This laid a basis for the evolvement of policies and programes in both education and nutrition.

TRANSITION TO LONGER-TERM OPERATION

In 1953 the words 'International' and 'Emergency' were dropped from the name, although the well established acronym was retained. The change was symbolic of a turning-point in UNICEF's policy—as from this date on, it became more involved in helping countries in designing and implementing longer-term activities and programmes in fields such as health, nutrition, and education. It was recognized that malnutrition, one of the major causes of mortality and morbidity in infants and young children, was not due only to lack of nutritious foods but also to various other factors including beliefs, taboos, and ignorance, and poor hygiene and sanitation, etc., which prevented and inhibited people from making full use of their resources. Hence, education became an integral part of the many community-based projects and concepts that evolved through the years and bore different names, such as Maternal and Child Health, Applied Nutrition, Mothercraft, Village Technology, and more recently Basic Services and Primary Health Care Projects. UNICEF in all of these efforts worked closely with other UN agencies, particularly the FAO and the WHO in nutrition and UNESCO in education; it also has had the advice and co-operation of the Protein Calorie Advisory Group and more recently the Sub-Committee on Nutrition of the United Nations Administrative Committee on Co-ordination.

A CHANGING ROLE IN SUPPLEMENTARY FEEDING

Soon after the change in UNICEF's general outlook in the early 1950s it became a matter of policy that, except under some emergency conditions, special educational activities should be an integral part of any supplementary feeding operations assisted by UNICEF. The distribution of milk-powder gradually became a minor part of UNICEF's assistance. Similarly, although UNICEF helped pioneer in the development of new lower-cost protein concentrates from oil seeds and fish, and nutritious mixtures containing them, the assistance to developing countries in the distribution of these products, especially those donated from outside, has been handled mainly by the World Food Programme, non-governmental organizations, and bilateral aid. With the increasing recognition of the special plight of young children, especially during the main weaning period, 6 months to 2 years of age, more emphasis was given to reaching this age group, including through channels in addition to MCH. When required in certain emergencies, UNICEF still provides selected foods and aids in their distribution.

UNICEF continues to co-operate with governments, through education and otherwise, to improve the effectiveness of supplementary feeding for the young children and pregnant and lactating women, regardless of the source of the food; where possible, the development of use of local resources is preferred. At the World Food Conference, Rome, 1974, the Executive Director of UNICEF, Mr Henry R. Labouisse, announced the 'basic services' approach, with selective supplementary feeding of the most needy, using local foods to the fullest extent possible, as part of that policy.

WORKING FOR NUTRITION IMPROVEMENT ON A BROADER FRONT

It became apparent as efforts of the earlier years were developing that for significant improvement in child nutrition an attack on a much broader scale was needed. Thus in 1957 the UNICEF Executive Board approved assistance within a programme of Expanded Aid to Nutrition, including surveys, training, education on child feeding and care, food fortification, etc. At about the same time, a special experimental programme of 'Nutrition Education and Related Activities' was launched, which mainly supported local production of nutritious foods combined with education on child feeding and care. Within a few years this programme, including the training of various types of worker required at all levels was being tried in many countries and came to be called 'Applied Nutrition'.

The experience with the latter approach has been mixed; the main contributions to success appear to be an appropriate involvement of the community at all stages, and understanding, encouragement, and support from government services at various levels. Nevertheless this basic approach to improvement of nutrition of poor people of the rural areas remains exceedingly important to this day, in parallel with large-scale programmes for production foods and as part of the efforts in rural development, provision of basic services and Primary Health Care.

TRAINING

For many years UNICEF has assisted with the training of various levels of personnel in the following categories: full-time nutrition workers, professionals and para-professionals who deal with nutrition in some of their work, and workers in various fields (health, agriculture, planning, etc.) who need nutrition orientation. Regional nutrition courses for both medical and non-medical personnel have been supported at various centres, including INCAP in Guatemala, the University of Ibadan in Nigeria, and the National Nutrition Institute of Hyderabad in India. UNICEF has co-operated in the injecting of human nutrition courses into the training programmes of agricultural and home science colleges and universities in India.

IMPROVEMENT OF NUTRITION THROUGH THE CHANNELS OF
FORMAL AND NON-FORMAL EDUCATION

By 1960 the UNICEF Executive Board was asking that more attention be given to the 'whole child' and all of the needs in child development, along with consideration of priorities for UNICEF assistance. Education was one of the selected areas.

A study for the 1977 UNICEF Board showed that UNICEF provides 20 per cent of outside assistance and 40 per cent of multilateral official aid in efforts to improve basic or other primary education. UNICEF's contribution is especially significant in promoting new ideas and experimentation.

In the frame of formal education programmes, UNICEF co-operates with governments in establishing goals to improve the quality of education, increase the number of its recipients, and especially to make sure that the type of education received is useful and adequate not only to provide alphabetization and formal teaching, but to help people resolve some of the practical problems they are faced with in their own communities, i.e. malnutrition, low food production, poor storage techniques, poor dietary habits, lack of hygiene, etc. Approximately one half of the 350 million children of primary-school age in developing countries are under UNICEF-assisted education projects. The importance of including the teaching of nutrition and home economics in the regular curriculum has been stressed, and implemented in many countries. The training of teachers for elementary and secondary schools is supported by UNICEF, these two topics are part of their training.

These new approaches (a considerable advance from the emergency book distribution and rehabilitation of damaged schools which was the main thrust in the late 1940s) have been developed in co-ordination with UNESCO and ILO with the aim of offering regular formal education and pre-vocational and vocational training to children, students, teachers, and supervisors emphasizing on the quality and relevance of education, especially geared to the community needs.

Non-formal education became a necessity in reaching those not covered by the formal education systems, including youths and adults who never had the opportunity of following formal education training and yet are both directly responsible for the welfare of their children and children-to-be, and are or should be active members of their communities. In the past few years programmes in non-formal education have been set up in co-operation with concerned governments in order to reach community dwellers. UNICEF has encouraged nutrition education within the non-formal education system—ranging from adult alphabetization to community-participation courses. It has also organized and supported many courses directed to elected village leaders and community-recruited village health workers, promoters, and auxiliaries, who, once trained, have the task of disseminating what they have learned to mothers and other community groups. Practical training is given in food demonstration, home and village gardening, small-animal rearing, use of purified water, hygiene, sanitation, etc.

PROJECT SUPPORT COMMUNICATIONS

UNICEF has developed a Project Support Communication network, which co-operates with governments in the spreading of information regarding health care, nutrition, education, community development, and other related fields, to the largest possible number of people in areas where UNICEF programmes are under way. This is done by supplying, or assisting in the development of, educational aids (for example: films, filmstrips, books, posters, etc.) and co-operating with various media. An example of Project Communication Support is to be found in Kenya. Beginning in 1975, educational information material (posters, manuals, pamphlets, etc.) has been developed while support and advice were given to various media to help disseminate certain educational messages. This is currently done through the press, in the form of articles and cartoons and through entertainment channels; for example, educational messages are being effectively interwoven with popular entertainment such as songs, plays, movies, puppet shows, and TV and radio soap operas. These shows have become very popular in Kenya.

In Mexico a project called PRODESH in the highlands of Chiapas undertook the responsibility of attacking a serious food shortage in the area, as well as a high incidence of malnutrition in vulnerable groups. In 1977 production of nutritious foods was promoted with the help of 316 male and female youth clubs with 6737 participants (of whom 41 per cent were women). Health village units were increased and training was provided for auxilliaries in which nutrition and nutrition education were strongly emphasized. In addition to programmes in health, education, agriculture, and women's participation, an innovative programme to support local food production called, 'Radio School Garden', is broadcast in four Mayan dialects and Spanish to peasants of remote villages, where promoters, trained with the help of UNICEF, give relevant explanations to youth clubs and peasant groups. The PRODESH educational communication department has strongly supported the programme and various audio-visual materials were produced including a special film. Project personnel and community leader's training and 538 primary schools, 5 agricultural technological schools, and 14 educational services are supported. Special training for schoolteachers in agriculture, health, and nutrition education is provided giving a multisectoral approach to the Basic Services strategy.

In Korea since 1968 the government's Applied Nutrition Project has been improving the life of rural communities in general and their nutritional status in particular and it has been actively supported by UNICEF, the FAO, and the WHO. UNICEF has supplied material and equipment to assist with baseline surveys, provincial nutrition laboratories, and village nutrition stations. It has also supported training activities and provided vehicles for supervision. UNICEF is continuing to support this project in the form of equipment, nutrition education grants, various kinds of training grants related to nutrition and consultant services, and will support the establishment of the Korean Institute for Nutrition Research and training and will promote the adoption of national foods and nutrition policies, with a principal focus on the requirements of vulnerable groups.

THE FUTURE

There are various indications that in the next decade or so there will be an increasing understanding of what needs to be done to improve nutrition, particularly in developing countries, and it is to be hoped there will also be an increasing will to make the necessary invest-ments. Establishment of effective educational elements in programmes to improve nutrition has been difficult, but this remains an essential challenge and opportunity for the future.

20 Nutrition education through health-care systems (WHO)

KALYAN BAGCHI

INTRODUCTION

Nutrition Education had participants from more than 60 countries speaks eloquently of the importance attributed to it as a means for combating malnutrition in the global context.

needs no emphasis. The fact that the International Conference on Nutrition Education had participants from more than 60 countries speaks eloquently of the importance attributed to it as a means for combating malnutrition in the global context.

Two distinct trends can now be noticed in the methodology of nutrition education. There are highly developed mass-communication techniques being employed, mostly by food industries, to promote food products under the umbrella of 'selling nutrition' in the developed countries. Most often the messages relate to the prevention of 'malnutrition of affluence', e.g. obesity, some types of cancer, coronary artery disease, hypertension, dental caries, etc. In recent years the replacement of breast-feeding by 'baby foods' is, to a large extent, due to the 'nutrition-oriented' high-pressure advertisements, which have deleterious results, at least in developing countries. Even in the United States, mass communication like television is used for messages 'negatively related to the nation's needs . . .' (Select Committee on Nutrition and Human Needs 1977). On the positive side, nutrition education in developed countries, through school curricula, can certainly go a long way in inducing desirable food habits. The recent decision in the United States to employ large-scale public nutrition education to reach the recent dietary goals is another positive example.

In the developing countries, the pattern of nutrition education is completely different. Only in a few cases is mass communication through television or radio adopted for educating the general population as a social-service measure (e.g. in Tanzania through the *Chakul ni Uhai*—'Food is Life'—Campaign) (WHO 1975). However, such use of mass media reaches only a very small fraction of the population, which badly needs such messages.

Among these vast, mostly rural under-serviced populations, nutrition education, wherever and whenever it permeates, is usually

given through one of the services such as health, community, or
rural development, women extension workers, or social welfare.
The methods are person-to-person or group communication. One
can say without hesitation that in most cases there is no clear idea
regarding methodology and impact. We are not even clear as to
whether we have succeeded or failed in such efforts and for what
reasons. The Eighth Report of the Joint FAO–WHO Expert Committee on Nutrition in 1971 rightly pointed out '. . .there is surprisingly little evidence that existing techniques of nutritional
education are effective or represent a good utilization of limited
resources, and it appears that some conventional programmes of
nutritional education have not succeeded in influencing food habits
in the desired manner'.

The purpose of this paper is to bring out some relevant facts about
nutrition education within this pattern, so far as they relate to the
health-care system in developing countries. The approach adopted in
the past, the present thinking, and the future strategies are discussed
and all these concern millions of malnourished, poverty-stricken,
mostly illiterate people living in areas where normal health and
social-services machinery scarcely permeates. Yet they are the vast
majority in most of the developing countries which need nutrition
education.

Nutrition education, as an intervention, came into prominence
with the realization that malnutrition, to a large extent, is due not
only to inadequate food availability, but also to faulty food habits,
some of them based on food prejudices, superstitions, and taboos.
The importance of nutrition education came into sharper focus when
investigations in various parts of the world revealed that undernutrition and malnutrition in the child population, especially the
protein-energy malnutrition with kwashiorkor and marasmus occupying the central position, were primarily due to faulty weaning. In
fact, since that time, nutrition education was accepted as an important measure for the promotion of child nutrition, and was included
as a routine procedure in maternal and child care. The Joint FAO–
WHO Expert Committee on Nutrition, with its first report in 1950,
started emphasizing the importance of nutrition education as a
nutrition promotion measure in the health sector. Since 1954,
education and training in nutrition have gained importance in the
programme of both the FAO and WHO. The fifth report of the
Joint FAO–WHO Expert Committee on Nutrition in 1958 stated
'Education in nutrition is a necessary part of practical programmes
to improve human nutrition. . .' The report further stated:

Education in nutrition can reach the people through various channels, of which the following are probably the most important:

(a) schools;
(b) maternal and child health and public health centres;
(c) community development and related programmes;
(d) agricultural and home-economics extension services.

Irrespective of the government sector or organization that implements nutrition education programmes, the aim is to produce certain changes in food consumption which are desirable for nutrition promotion. One should note that the efforts of nutrition education are mostly directed towards changes in food consumption and do not, in most cases, give emphasis to other factors which interfere with the consumption and biological utilization of food.

NUTRITION EDUCATION ACTIVITIES IN THE HEALTH SECTOR

It would be worthwhile to trace the development of nutrition education activities in the health sector. With the realization that malnutrition is a health problem and that the health sector should take some measures for its amelioration, the pattern of health sector intervention for prevention purposes during the early phase was the following:

(1) assessment of the malnutrition problem, mostly through surveys based on clinical signs and symptoms and supported by food consumption surveys;
(2) distribution of vitamin and mineral tablets, mostly obtained as aid from international or bilateral bodies;
(3) distribution of milk powder, again mostly from the same sources; and
(4) nutrition education of mothers attending the maternal and child care centres.

Possibly, the reasons why nutrition education was very commonly adopted as an intervention measure, not only by the health sector but also by other sectors or organizations, were:

(1) no significant capital investment was needed;
(2) no highly trained professionals were considered necessary;
(3) there was flexibility regarding the infrastructure, e.g. school-house, rural club, health centres, or even individual village homes; and
(4) there was an erroneous impression that the food habits can be changed easily by 'lecturing'. The main reason for the relative lack of evaluation was the 'taken-for-granted' attitude towards the impact of nutrition education.

Plus points for the health sector

There are additional reasons as to why nutrition education programmes became more acceptable to the health sector, the principal ones being:

1. The health infrastructures like maternal and child health (MCH) clinics or health centres always have a sizeable number of subjects (as patients), especially women, to whom educational messages can be conveyed. In other words, no difficulty is experienced in getting an 'audience' for the educational session.

2. There is no difficulty in motivating the subjects, unlike the situation in similar programmes in other sectors. Mothers attending the health centres or clinics with sick children are highly motivated to 'learn' for the sake of their children.

3. The educators (in the case of health sectors, the health professionals), again, unlike similar workers in many other sectors, are respected by the people. In fact they enjoy a high credibility. A health visitor or midwife going on her home visits is a much wanted and respected person. Workers in many other sectors have to establish their credibility with the villages, which is not always an easy task.

4. The base or the infrastructure needed for such sessions is conveniently present in the health sector, e.g. health centres, maternal and child care clinics, nutrition rehabilitation centres, etc.

Common defects

In spite of the two main advantages, viz. the comparative ease in getting the locations and subjects for education sessions, and the fairly high acceptability of the educators, nutrition education activity in the health sector was rarely taken seriously as an important task— and in most instances was included as a routine low-priority activity conducted in a perfunctory manner. While clinical work was supervised, nutrition education was only rarely supervised. A common pattern emerged in which the main defects were:

(1) most often the messages to be conveyed to the mothers were imparted in the form of 'teaching' and invariably there were too many (the *educators 'taught' what they 'learnt'*);
(2) most often the messages, for the reasons mentioned above, were of a textbook pattern for developed countries, e.g. 'basic five or seven groups for balanced diet' and going frequently into discussions about nutrients (protein, vitamins, etc.) well beyond the understanding of the audience;
(3) the health workers who acted as educators quite often were ignorant of the cultural basis for food practices in the area, and ther ˉ re offered advice which clashed with these;
(4) being clinically oriented, the educators usually regarded nutrition education as something vague, in contrast to the clear-cut clinical work with its visible results. Moreover, an overburdened health worker in a health centre or a clinic regarded nutrition education as an additional and rather undesirable load.

A typical scene of nutrition education in the health sector

Possibly old memories will be revived if a typical education session is described. Even now the same scene is re-enacted in many countries in various types of health infrastructures. A typical scene is found in the out-patient clinics of a health centre or an antenatal or postnatal clinic of an MCH centre. A nutrition education session is conducted in one such overcrowded clinic, or in a separate room nearby. The audience are the mothers waiting to be called in for examination. In other words the waiting time is utilized with the idea of 'filling-the-gap'. The attention of the audience is not on what is being discussed, but on the delay in being called. The educator very often is a nurse, midwife, or a health visitor, who regards this responsibility as an additional load, and discharges this by giving a lecture, with the help of some food models or charts. Sometimes cooking demonstrations are given with cooking utensils and gadgets mostly unfamiliar to the mothers. Follow-up of the subjects to ascertain the effect of such education is rarely done. Messages, which are too many, are invariably based on the nutrient content of foods, on food groups, and on how to plan a balanced diet.

Stages of rationalization

With the gradual development of health education activities and programmes, nutrition education, especially in the health sector, was more rationalized, undergoing significant procedural changes of which two were quite important:

(1) Nutrition education was recognized as a part of health education. In other words, it was realized that, without simultaneous measures for health promotion, education on correct food habits would produce marginal effects.
(2) Well-designed and tested media were gradually employed instead of just 'lecturing'. Thus flip-charts, flannelgraphs, etc. were designed and used for nutrition education.

The real impetus to nutrition education was given with the introduction of applied nutrition programmes, sponsored by UNICEF with the collaboration of the FAO and WHO in several developing countries during the sixties. For the first time, nutrition education to promote satisfactory food practices was placed on an equal footing with that of food production. Creating nutrition awareness was regarded as a motivating factor behind home and kitchen gardens. Nutrition and health education was not only regarded as the responsibility of the health sector, but was also included as an essential component of education on home-making, conducted by women extension workers of the community or rural development sector, and through school education. A noticeable defect was that numerous and diverse messages were conveyed to the same subjects through these sectors during the same period, and in several cases, as a result or a lack of co-ordination among the sectors, the messages were conflicting. In many countries, as part of the Applied Nutrition Project, considerable interest and activities were directed towards production of nutrition education media and materials.

Other internationally or bilaterally aided programmes in many countries—mass feeding programmes—provided support to nutrition education in varying degrees. In most of the skimmed-milk feeding programmes, however, nutrition education was hardly conducted at all. In subsequent years, school-meal programmes in a large number of countries had important components of nutrition education. The education was more through the meal provided, although formal education in the school curriculum was also adopted, usually through health, hygiene, or home-science teachers. In recent years feeding programmes supported by the World Food Programme have quite often health and nutrition education components built into them. However, how effectively these are carried out in the midst of such terribly busy activity as the Feeding Programme is not yet clear. Its impact is more difficult to ascertain, and rarely has the impact been evaluated. Moreover, in quite a few of these programmes, unknown foods not available locally are promoted and in the long run these have no positive educational impact.

Nutrition rehabilitation centres: a medium for nutrition education

While searching for instances where nutrition education has been effective, one must admit that possibly a good example is nutrition rehabilitation centres, where nutrition education is imparted in the most rationalized form. The main plus points are the following.

1. In the usual nutrition-education programmes, the common practice is to convey messages about desirable changes in food consumption —*desirable from the point of view of educators*, that is! As for the mothers, there is nothing that they can see that will convince them of the benefit of the desired changes. In the nutrition rehabilitation centres, the mothers who stay with their children not only know about the desired changes in food habits, but they also observe their sick children being rehabilitated through the desired change in food consumption.

2. The mothers, i.e. the target group for education, are fully involved in the selection, preparation, and handling of food. They see food hygiene in practice. They are not casual one-day observers, such as

those who attend quite often 'under pressure', as in the case of nutrition education through other health bases like health centres and clinics.

It is not surprising that nutrition education through nutrition rehabilitation centres produced much better results. In several follow-up studies it was found that children of mothers who had been in such centres rarely came back to the centres with severe malnutrition. The nutritional status of the siblings of children whose mothers who were once admitted to such rehabilitation centres was always found to be better than other children in the neighbourhood. Obviously the mothers were putting into practice what they had learnt during their stay in the centre, for their other children who had not been admitted to the centre.

However, even with nutrition rehabilitation centres, the impact of nutrition education is not as strong as one expects. An extensive evaluation, made by Beaudry-Darismé and Latham (1973) of nutrition rehabilitation centres, revealed that the nutrition-education component is relatively weak. Several reasons have been ascribed for this, of which the following are important:

(1) The staff of the centres had a tendency to regard curative aspects as much more important than the 'preventive' work, of which nutrition education is a component. 'Most health personnel find it more satisfying, and believe that it is more humanitarian to devote their energy to curing diseases rather than promoting health.'

(2) Quite often the mothers who stayed with their children in the centres were regarded as outsiders to be utilized for relieving some of the work-load of the regular staff.

(3) Educational materials for mothers were too often set at an unnecessarily high level, and the mothers failed to absorb them. Sometimes, unrealistic messages were conveyed, e.g. examples of desired foods given were outside the economic reach of most mothers.

(4) Fathers were not involved at any stage in such education processes.

It is interesting to note that most of these factors operate, with adverse effects, in other health-care systems as well, e.g. in health centres and in clinics. The health workers need a thorough orientation before they can overcome these drawbacks. The content and the methodology of nutrition education, even after years of implementation, remains in many cases extremely confusing. However, this should not detract us from the value of such activity as a major approach to community nutrition problems; possibly the only active nutrition intervention in the most peripheral areas in most countries.

Through these trials and errors nutrition education programmes, as they are now at their present stage, can benefit greatly from three simple lessons learnt through years of experience:

(1) messages can be conveyed much more effectively through simple well-tested media;
(2) a few realistic and simple messages are quickly absorbed; and
(3) the educator would be aware of the culture and food habits of the population among whom nutrition education is to be conducted.

HOW FAR HAS THE PROGRAMME BEEN EFFECTIVE—EVALUATIONS?

Nutrition education, though widely adopted as a nutrition intervention measure, has been evalutated very infrequently. The value of any nutrition-education programme lies in the extent to which it produces the desired changes. It is, therefore, surprising that so little work has been done to test whether such programmes have achieved the objectives. With a little consideration, one can identify the probable reasons:

1. *The difficulty in evaluating nutrition education programmes.* The important question asked, and which is even now being asked, is 'What should be the indicators for evaluation?' If the indicator is the result of a better consumption, i.e. the improved nutritional status, then we must remember that this is influenced by a number of non-dietary factors as well. To what extent can the improved status be ascribed to the effects of nutrition education alone? Should the indicators be nutrition awareness, or change in attitude, or change in practices, then we must keep in mind that these are difficult to measure and correlate only with education. An example in recent years clarified this attitude towards evaluation.

The Applied Nutrition Programme, sponsored by UNICEF in collaboration with the FAO and WHO, was evaluated in several countries. While considering the production component, the indicators were easily identified as the number of kitchen gardens, the family units with poultry farms, etc. Evaluation of nutrition training components was similarly easy on the basis of training courses and the number of people trained. When it came to the question of evaluating the nutrition education component, the matter had to be dropped since no suitable parameters were identified. There was reluctance, quite justifiably, to use health parameters like height and weight of the child population. This situation applied to most nutrition education projects or programmes when it came to evaluation.

2. *The absence of a simple method for evaluation.* This is, no

doubt, an important limitation. The Office of Nutrition of the Agency for International Development of the United States brought out a field-guide for the evaluation of nutrition education in 1975. The Agency very rightly states in the Preface that there is an 'absence of an accepted and tried evaluation methodology which is simple to apply'. However, one must admit that even this 'simple' methodology developed by AID would hardly be suitable for assessing the effectiveness of such programmes. The input needed for the evaluation is impossible to collect at the level where such education is conducted. It should be made clear at this stage, that evaluation of various categories has been done on nutrition education carried out through mass-communication media, especially in the developed countries. The effect on food habits of high powered commercial advertisements through mass media like television and radio in the developed countries is well known and adequately documented.

The subjective impression regarding the effects of nutrition can be broadly divided into two categories, of two extremes. At one extreme is the opinion that significant dietary changes can be made—and relatively easily—by education, and this is reflected by significant changes in nutritional status, e.g. increase in heights and weights of children and even some biochemical parameters like haemoglobin. At the other extreme, is the impression that is is difficult to change food habits by nutrition education alone. Knowledge and attitude can be changed to some extent but the change of actual dietary practices is difficult and time-consuming. Possibly, the real state would be in between the two extremes.

FUTURE STRATEGY—LESSONS LEARNT

A big question can be posed now—'Are we in a position to plan future strategy in nutrition education, knowing that there are not many lessons to learn from evaluation?' The answer, as far as it relates to the health-care system, is yes—with the provision that efforts should be made to analyse critically our past efforts, which might not be strictly according to the usual evaluation protocols, and to learn which factors led to success in some projects, and at the same time identify the factors which were possible causes of failure.

The WHO's attention is mainly directed towards developing strategies through which countries can make nutrition services available to people who are in need of them. With the realization that primary health care—appropriate health care to the maximum number of people—is the only solution at present to provide the much needed health care to all, the WHO strategy is to incorporate nutrition activities into the primary health-care services and with any other services that reach the ultimate periphery. Nutrition education has to be built in within this framework, occupying an important place among nutrition intervention. The WHO is now currently engaged in making a review of all experiences to know how best we can utilize this measure.

Analysis of underlying factors

The pattern of malnutrition in the developing countries gives an indication of the approach through which nutrition education gives better dividends. With the virtual disappearance of obvious deficiency diseases like beriberi and scurvy, undernutrition and protein energy malnutrition dominate the global scene of malnutrition. The major victims are children under five years, and pregnant and lactating women. These two facts, which indicate the nature of the problem and the age-groups affected, will be of crucial importance in developing strategy.

It would be useful to make a tentative analysis and try to identify the adverse factors—direct and indirect—which cause malnutrition. Obviously nutrition education will have to be directed in such a way as to prevent these factors or to mitigate their effects. By and large, these factors are:

(1) highly inadequate diet on which the malnourished pregnant women live and then deliver small 'at-risk' babies (both mothers and babies are vulnerable);
(2) early stoppage of breast-feeding or its substitution by artificial feeding, which is not only nutritionally inadequate but leads to gastroenteritis;
(3) breast-feeding continued for one to one-and-a-half years without introducing supplementary foods from five or six months;
(4) delayed or defective sharing of the family diet after complete weaning;
(5) failure to use suitable available foods in the most advantageous manner;
(6) high incidence of infectious diseases, especially gastroenteritis, precipitating malnutrition in children who were on the border-line;
(7) lack of environmental sanitation, especially the absence of safe water; and
(8) repeated closely spaced pregnancies leading to maternal malnutrition and the birth of small 'at-risk' babies who have no nutritional reserve and who are highly susceptible to nutritional deficiencies.

Undoubtedly there are many other minor factors, varying from place to place. However, the ones mentioned above can be regarded as more or less a model of the causes of malnutrition in most developing countries.

Education for nutrition improvement

It stands to reason that education for nutrition improvement (rather than nutrition education) should be broadly summarized under the following categories:

(1) education for promotion and protection of breast-feeding, for introduction of supplementary feeding, and for weaning;

(2) education on the most advantageous use of available foods;

(3) education on food hygiene and on environmental sanitation; and

(4) education for birth spacing.

It is obvious that education conducted under one category will produce a very limited impact, and in certain circumstances no impact at all.

Having established the broad areas in which education has to be imparted for an overall improvement of nutrition health, it is important to describe the factors which would determine the logistics of such an activity.

— Who are the audience? They are mostly illiterate people, living in predominantly rural areas, with deep-rooted food practices and not exposed to any extraneous influences which might modify their food habits or exposed to the wrong ones through commercial advertisements.

— Their health and nutritional status, especially their children's, are extremely low. Malnutrition and infectious diseases, especially gastroenteritis, are the usual pattern.

— Economically they are mostly below the poverty line. They have no economic means to make a significant addition to their diet. In most instances, the availability of food is also greatly limited.

— They have no or very little access to h alth or social services since the infrastructures of these services do not usually reach the peripheral areas.

Logistics

What should be the logistics under these circumstances? The most vital step is to identify the services or personnel who operate at the periphery. This will of course vary from one country to another. In most developing countries peripheral areas are not covered by any form of health service. The present strategy of the WHO, to cover these populations by primary health care, is possibly the best available solution at the moment. Several countries are experimenting with similar or slightly modified strategies with the same objective.

Irrespective of the strategy, the burden of health care in the peripheral part of most developing countries will be on a single worker, a multipurpose worker, who will of necessity have to do minimum curative work and as much preventive work as possible. This lone worker—a primary health care worker, or health auxiliary, health aide, medical assistant, or whatever name given to them—will have to undertake nutrition education along with other responsibilities.

Several points emerge as corollaries:

1. There is no specialization in services or education at this level, since the health-worker is the only person giving treatment. The broad educational strategy described before with components of nutrition, communicable disease control, family planning, etc., can very conveniently be done by him.

2. Since this multipurpose worker is loaded with various responsibilities, the educational part should be designed to occupy as little time as possible. The messages to be chosen should be few and the vital ones. For example, in the field of infant and child nutrition, the two following messages, carried out forcefully, can do wonders:

> (a) promotion and protection of breast-feeding, with some foods from the family diet, from five or six months, for supplementation; and
> (b) teaching that the correct way to wean the child is with foods which are locally available and acceptable and normally used in the family diet (for example, in most areas, a mixture of cereals and legumes is normally used).

3. The messages should be as simple as possible. The training of multipurpose workers should be so designed that they in turn can convey the same messages to the subjects in a comprehensible manner.

4. Irrespective of the government sector to which the peripheral workers belong, their training for conducting nutrition education should receive special consideration. The usual practice of imparting textbook-type conventional scientific discussion of nutrition should be replaced by task-oriented nutrition, indicating clearly the relationship with other related activities. Some examples will clarify this point. Gastroenteritis is an important precipitator of malnutrition and is most commonly associated with it. The role of nutrition educators will be first to educate the mother as to how to prevent dehydration, or to correct it if already present, and then gradually rehabilitate by food intake. In the normal nutrition training oral rehydration has no place. Similarly, the cause and consequence of malnutrition and too frequent closely spaced pregnancies should be emphasized in education.

Needless to say, this comprehensive approach to nutrition education does not apply only to the health sector, but also with equal force to workers of other sectors responsible for nutrition and child care. Nutrition education, in the present context of existing situations in developing countries, would better be interpreted as 'education for nutrition improvement'.

REFERENCES

Beaudry-Darisme, M. and Latham, M. (1973). Nutrition rehabilitation centres: an evaluation of their performance. *J. trop. Paed. Env. cld Hlth* 19, p. 299.

FAO–WHO (1971). *The eighth report of the FAO–WHO Committee on Nutrition.*

Office of Nutrition, Technical Assistance Bureau, Agency for Technical Development (1975). *A field guide for evaluation of nutrition education.*

Select Committee on Nutrition and Human Needs, US Senate (1977). *Dietary goals for the United States.*

WHO (1975). *Report of the interregional workshop on nutrition in family health, Morogoro, Tanzania.* WHO document NUT76.1.

21 Nutrition education in the Republic of Korea

MICHAEL PARK

Nutrition education usually has a dramatic pay-off among adults as well as children at any income level. Ignorance about the nutritional value of local foods, misconceptions about the appropriateness of certain diets for vulnerable groups, and traditional food-allocation patterns within the family are all causes of undernutrition. The World Health Organization estimates that one-half or more of the nutritional problems of Africa, for example, could be solved through appropriate education.

Nutrition education reaching the home and capable of being applied in family food patterns is the ultimate road to good nutrition. It should be practical and applied, adapted to economic and agricultural possibilities and it can be an invaluable part of community development, both in urban and rural areas. To evolve an effective nutrition education programme, community participation is imperative. Involving people in the community in planning this programme is one way of enlisting their active support on a project.

The ways of achieving successful nutrition education are, first to obtain the interest and involvement of decision-makers and problem-solving administrative level personnel, secondly encourage co-ordination among the government ministries concerned, thirdly to stimulate the active participation and involvement of the community concerned, and fourthly to train workers at the grass-roots level.

Nutrition education should be the subject of a separate plan of work or action programme in a properly planned nutrition project, and it should be an on-going programme with proper sequence and development, and periodic evaluation.

NUTRITION EDUCATION THROUGH FORMAL SCHOOL EDUCATION

The school system in Korea follows the pattern of elementary school (six years), middle school (three years), high school (three years), and college or university (four years). Exceptions to this rule are two-year junior college and six-year medical colleges. Compulsory education begins for all children at the age of six years in elementary school.

Nutrition education through schools is of particular importance because of its profound influence on the coming generation's ideas about foods and nutrition and hygiene. Therefore co-operation with schools and the education departments is essential at all levels.

The Ministry of Education and the Korea Education Development Institute (KEDI) have developed a syllabus on nutrition subjects which integrates nutrition and population education in the schools. The high-school girls are required to take the subject of home economics, including food and nutrition; and the subject of housekeeping —which covers nutrition—is an elective subject for middle-school girls.

The Departments of Food and Nutrition in colleges are teaching nutrition education with a revised curriculum, and a qualification in this subject is required in order to become a dietician. In Korea ninety-two schools—universities, colleges, junior colleges, technical colleges, and special correspondence colleges—offer courses in home economics and nutrition, and some 15 000 students enter these departments each year. All home-economics programmes include nutrition education.

The courses of applied-nutrition/community-nutrition have been newly introduced into the advanced home-economics and nutrition programme for MS and Ph.D degrees.

NUTRITION EDUCATION THROUGH RADIO SCHOOLS

Junior College

The Korea Junior College of the Air and Correspondence (KOJUCAC) was established in 1972 as a two-year junior college attached to Seoul National University. A main objective of the college is to enhance the educational level of Koreans by providing new opportunities for higher education for those youths and adults who are unable to attend regular colleges and universities. The college is fully accredited by the Ministry of Education, and its graduates can enter regular four-year colleges and universities if they pass the Government-administered qualification examinations.

The college has five departments: Home Economics; Agriculture; Elementary Education; Business Management; and Public Administration. The total number of students to be admitted is set at 12 000, including 2000 for the Home Economics Department, per year. Students are selected according to their high-school academic records, the admission quota assigned to each province, and the applicants' current occupations in relation to the proposed field of study.

The methods of instruction and evaluation consist of four major areas and these are: (1) students' self-study, with text materials specially prepared by the college; (2) radio instruction—listening to radio lectures consisting of three 15-minute programmes a week for two years over the national network of the Korean Broadcasting System; (3) submission of assigned reports to the college faculty for evaluation; (4) schooling at the co-operating institutions (six national universities and sixteen colleges) for four weeks per year.

A total of 87 credits, 66 credits in Home Economics and 21 for General Education, is required for graduation, and about 30 per cent of the Home Economics curriculum is related to nutrition and food studies, e.g. Basic Nutrition, Special Nutrition, Food and Food Preparation, Meal Planning and Management, Food Science. Some 70 per cent of the home-economics students are elementary-school teachers, and there are also nurses, home-economics extension workers, family-planning workers, social-welfare workers, cooks, and teachers in kindergarten or day-care centres.

High schools

According to the 1975 census, some two million Koreans between the ages of 15 and 34 have completed middle school only. In spite of a rapid growth in the number of schools at all levels, approximately 30 per cent of middle-school graduates are not admitted to high school each year. As an attempt to provide high school education to this large population, the Air and Correspondence High School programme was developed in Korea in March 1974.

Forty existing regular high schools, 8 in Seoul and 32 in other cities, were selected for the radio and correspondence education programme, and it will be expanded to other cities throughout the country in 1977–8. As of April 1976 the total number of students in the programme has been 18 800 and about 70 per cent of the students have occupations.

The methods of instruction are the same as the junior college mentioned above. A textbook of home economics—including food and nutrition—for the girl students was prepared by the university home economists.

NUTRITION EDUCATION THROUGH THE APPLIED NUTRITION PROJECT

The Applied Nutrition Project (ANP) in Korea was initiated as a part of the rural development programme to improve the life of rural communities and their nutritional status in 1968, and it has been supported by UNICEF, the FAO, and the WHO. UNICEF has supplied materials and equipment for nutrition centres and village nutrition stations. It also supported training activities and provided vehicles for supervision. Since 1974 the ANP, organized and operated by the Office of Rural Development, has started collaboration with the

Ministry of Education and with the Ministry of Health.

Pilot school-garden and school nutrition education programmes organized by the Ministry of Education, and the orientation-training in nutrition for health personnel under the Ministry of Health and Social Affairs, are important parts of the project. This is a thriving and stimulating project, which is forming close links with the national Saemaul Movement (New Community Movement).

The Korean ANP has placed as much emphasis on nutrition education as on an improved standards of living. It is thus a combination that is synergistic and highly successful. Nutrition education will continue to be a fundamental and continuous village-level activity, including food preparation, dissemination of new recipes, etc. The production and distribution of nutrition-education materials for village-level activities and for training are the responsibility of the Office of Rural Development. The Office of Rural Development has produced nutrition-education materials, e.g. films, slides, books, pamphlets, leaflets, posters, in its well equipped audio-visual laboratories.

Concentrated guidance was given to 1047 pilot and 138 voluntary ANP villages which have 'village nutrition stations' equipped with various cooking utensils. The main functions of the nutrition station are cooking demonstration and practice, food processing and preservation of local foodstuffs, group feeding during farming seasons, child feeding at seasonal day-care centres, and nutrition education.

Some 400 Home Improvement and Applied Nutrition Project workers at central, provincial, and county levels have trained over two million villagers at the meetings, more than twice a month, of the Villager Women's Home Improvement Clubs. The main subjects for training have been food production, food preparation, processing and preservation, nutritional care for vulnerable groups, balanced diet, instructions for using food processing equipment, etc.

Three nutrition-education vans of the Office of Rural Development visit remote areas to provide extension services including nutrition education.

SCHOOL-LUNCH PROGRAMME AND SCHOOL-GARDEN/NUTRITION EDUCATION

The school lunch programme in Korea was initiated by UNICEF for relief purpose in 1953, after the Korean War, and it was assisted by CARE and USAID until 1973. The Ministry of Education established various pilot projects and programmes to study the most economical method of developing a nation-wide, community-supported school-lunch and nutrition education programme at the elementary school level. The Ministry has developed new approaches for the elementary-school-lunch programmes emphasizing nutrition education and training, community participation, and school/community food production.

There are three types of school-lunch programme in Korea. These are, first a protective feeding programme for 470 000 needy children living in offshore, remote, and urban slum areas. Secondly a recipient funded programme for 810 000 children; and thirdly a self-sufficient feeding programme for 46 000 children of 21 urban and 55 rural schools. Some 1.3 million schoolchildren are now participating in the school-lunch programmes, out of a total 5.5 million elementary school children in Korea. The Government will provide US$ 7.3 million for the school-lunch programme during 1977.

Nutrition training and education for personnel involved in school-lunch/nutrition-education programmes, including schoolteachers and community representatives, was conducted, and the curriculum of the training course included subjects of basic nutrition, food production, food preparation, sanitation, and food hygiene. Besides the theoretical lectures, the workship participants took field trips for practical exercises. The schoolteachers deliver nutrition messages to the children during the lunch time, and the parents of the schoolchildren attend lectures on nutrition education twice a year.

UNICEF has provided demonstration garden equipment for 55 pilot schools in the school-garden/nutrition-education programme, for self-sufficient lunch programmes, and nutrition training grants for 760 persons in the fields of food production and preparation of the schools.

NUTRITION TRAINING OF HEALTH PERSONNEL

The specific function of health-education specialists in government services is to advise health personnel on how to make health education, including nutrition education, effective, but most of them have insufficient background-training and lack the specialized knowledge of Korean educational techniques.

Special training activities under the auspices of the Ministry of Health and Social Affairs were therefore organized for 210 'nutrition guidance workers', mainly public health nurses and midwives at health centres, in order to improve their knowledge of food and nutrition, and UNICEF provided financial assistance for the one-week training courses during 1976. The Ministry has developed the text for nutrition training of health personnel, which includes the subjects of basic nutrition, child and maternal nutrition, food preparation, national nutrition surveys, nutrition education at school and in the community, and applied nutrition. Following the completion of their studies, both theoretical and practical, they were asked to pass a simple test to determine their new level of capability in the subject.

The Korea Health Development Institute (KHDI) has selected three pilot areas for developing a low-cost general health delivery system for the rural population. Pre-service training is under action with the newly developed curriculum, including community nutrition education for the selected nurses who will be served as village health workers.

The Public Health Department of the Korean Red Cross has developed health-education materials, and it has already produced ten sets of audio-visual materials, using colour slides together with sound recordings on health and nutrition topics. The Peace Corps volunteers in Korea are also developing health and nutrition education materials for rural people.

NUTRITION EDUCATION THROUGH THE MASS MEDIA

The voluntary agencies—including CARE—provided assistance to the Ministry of Health and Social Affairs for a nutrition education programme through the mass media in 1970. Two 30-second nutrition spot-messages per day and 20-minute dramas on nutrition education on Saturdays were broadcast by the Government broadcasting system for one year. Various printed materials on nutrition education were distributed through health centres, day-care centres, women's clubs, and other appropriate outlets.

During 1976 nutrition education for farmers was broadcast 59 times through the nation-wide network of the national radio and TV system. The Office of Rural Development also publishes an *Agricultural Technical Bulletin* which includes articles on food and nutrition.

Broadcasting systems, one government and four private, in Korea have offered programmes on housekeeping including food and nutrition education, and TV programmes offer the same programme frequently. In addition to the radio and TV nutrition programmes, newspapers and magazines have recently become active by inserting articles on food and nutrition in the publications.

But more active participation of the mass media is required to enhance nutrition education for the general public. According to a recent study report, 49.6 per cent of the 16 253 women who visited the Red Cross Blood Institute in Seoul were found to be unsuitable for blood donation, with 74.2 per cent of the unqualified donors suffering from anaemia. The main causes of the anaemia in women are unbalanced diet to control their weight, menstruation, breast-feeding, pregnancy, and the traditional prejudice against Korean women which requires them to serve the most nutritious dishes only to men. It is necessary to present effective scientific information on food and nutrition through the mass media to improve the nutrition education of the public.

INTEGRATED NUTRITION EDUCATION PROGRAMMES IN
DAY-CARE CENTRES

Nutrition education should include effective demonstration of the main facts about nutrition, and sometimes the supplementary feeding of vulnerable groups, as well as practice by the mothers in food preparation.

A main purpose of this project is to integrate supplementary feeding for pre-school children, nutrition education, and family planning into a comprehensive effort to improve family life. This programme has been conducted through the day-care centres with the joint assistance from the Ministry of Health and Social Affairs, the World Food Programme, and CARE in Korea. The day-care centres are serving lunch and snacks to the children and giving instructions to the mothers whose children are attending the centres on supplementary feeding, hygienic preparation of foods with minimum loss of nutrients, and other subjects on food and nutrition.

22 The introduction of nutrition education in primary schools and in adult education

F.D.S. NGEGBA

Under the auspices of the Bununbu Project, 'Training of Primary School Teachers for Rural Areas', an attempt is being made to introduce and strengthen nutrition education in the primary school curriculum and adult education programmes in the rural areas in Sierra Leone. This effort arises from the need to arrest the growing incidence of under- and malnutrition, the resultant growth retardation, and the high rates of (especially infant) mortality in the rural areas. This situation is due mainly to ignorance and the overriding influence of tradition and superstition.

The approach adopted is integration involving the school and its curriculum on the one hand, and the community—parents, guardians, voluntary organizations, out-of-school youths and bilateral agencies through non-formal education—on the other hand.

THE SCHOOL AND ITS CURRICULUM

Attempts are being made to develop an integrated primary-school curriculum with a rural-biased core and optional components emphasizing urban learning needs. These are being tried experimentally in twenty selected primary schools with a 20-mile radius of Bunumbu college. In these curriculum exercises the co-operation of all teachers in the twenty schools is actively enlisted through week-end workshops conducted at the College. In addition to the Home Economics Curriculum being the special responsibility of the Department, the UNESCO expert and her counterpart actively co-operate with the primary-school teachers and other College staff in working out the curriculum in other subjects to ensure the inclusion of nutrition education. Thus materials have already been developed, for example in agriculture, to help children participate in food production, which is used in the schools' feeding programmes. Instructional materials and procedures in agricultural education include practical experiments to determine the effect of nutrients on the successful growth and development of plants. From these experiments relevant analogies are drawn to demonstrate that just as plants require certain nutrients for proper growth and development, so do human beings require certain nutrients for healthy growth and development. This idea is then reflected in the Home Economics programme in lessons on the value of vitamins, proteins, minerals, and other nutrients to human growth and development.

Similarly, in the Art and Basic Crafts Department, posters are prepared to illustrate the effects of the deficiency of certain nutrients on plant and human growth and development. Posters and other illustrative materials are also made to illustrate the seasonal and regional availability of local foodstuffs and are used in Geography and Adult Education classes. In Language Arts stories, simple poems, rhymes, and songs based on nutrition are written with the aid of the teachers, thus instructions on nutrition are given indirectly through other subjects in the integrated curriculum.

The care of the body and the hygienic preparation of foods are included in the syllabuses of physical and health education in the Primary School. Under the supervision of the home economics teacher children actually participate in the preparation of local food items produced by themselves in the school's agricultural and day-feeding programmes. These practical exercises provide the link between home economics and nutrition on the one hand and agriculture and health education on the other hand.

NON-FORMAL ADULT EDUCATION

Through parent–teacher associations and by means of other direct contacts with the school, such as adult education classes, parents and guardians receive informal lessons in nutrition education, and are encouraged to visit the school occasionally and to see their children at work. At convenient times, women from the village are invited to the school to participate in food-preparation lessons and exercises along with their children under the guidance of the home economics teacher. One advantage of this is the resulting cross-fertilization of ideas whereby traditional methods with proven value are taught to the children while the local women have the opportunity of participation in the 'modern' methods of the school. For this purpose, women student-teachers have been admitted into the College and they are receiving specialized training to enable them to work well in an integrated situation. This approach underscores the 'community school' concept which is the underlying philosophy of our programme.

Multidisciplinary Community Development Councils have been organized by the teachers in each school area under College staff supervision, and these augment the contact between the school and the community. Schoolrooms vacated by the children at the end of the school day are being used for adult education classes. As part of adult instructional exercises, especially in adult literacy classes, follow-up readers and posters prepared by the school as referred to above are translated into the vernacular language, and these contain elements of nutritional instruction and other allied disciplines. As well as these, practical demonstration lessons are included to dispel traditional prejudices, for example children are precluded from eating meat or fish or drinking milk, as these are believed to cause worm infections in children.

These instructions are buttressed by structured in-service education for teachers and other community leaders to sensitize them to community problems and needs and the new methodology developed at the College for combating them. In these in-service education programmes, the co-operation of other sectoral Ministries, voluntary organizations, and bilateral agencies is sought and fully utilized. Seminars and discussion groups form part of the programme.

It is as yet not possible to evaluate the effects of these programmes. Careful observation and documentation are being done. As part of their projects, student teachers are encouraged to develop an interest in the community and in the children in the villages, and to observe and document changes in nutritional and other behaviour resulting from the implementation of our programmes. These findings will eventually be analysed and interpreted and modifications made in our programmes as part of the evaluative process.

23 A regional centre for nutrition education in Guatemala

SUSANA ICAZA

BACKGROUND

Before 1966, the five countries of Central America and Panama had no more than 30 nutritionists responsible for all their public-health nutrition programmes and institutional food services. In one of these countries there was only one nutritionist. The possibilities for each country to create and implement its own school of nutrition were more than remote. A feasible solution to this problem, therefore, was to create a regional school attached to one of the national universities of the area which could provide professional training to students from the six countries. This is how, in January 1966, the School of Nutrition of the Institute of Nutrition of Central America and Panama (INCAP), in Guatemala, initiated its educational activities with the first group of students.

PURPOSES OF THE SCHOOL

There were two main purposes which guided the foundation of the School:

(1) to train nutritionist-dietitians for the countries of Central America and Panama where need for their services was badly felt; and
(2) to serve as a model for a regional centre of nutrition education at the college level.

METHODS

A four-year study and work curriculum was developed, covering all areas related to the nutrition of the individual, the family, and the community. First-year courses deal with fundamental knowledge in the basic sciences. Second-year studies emphasize fundamental knowledge in nutrition. Courses included in the third year of studies are aimed at providing students with the essentials required for the application of nutrition in programmes directed to the individual, the institution, and the community.

Along with regular classes, educational experiences are carefully planned so as to include active participation of the students in meetings, seminars, and Central American nutrition congresses. Visits to other institutions allow them also to observe various types of programme, as well as to collect data related to the subject-matter of their regular courses. Public offices, hospitals, and institutional food services are the main sources of this type of information.

Students, too, must undertake numerous teaching activities. Elementary and secondary schools, as well as institutions of higher education, are essential elements in their learning process. These serve both as subjects of inquiry and as fields of practice for the development of teaching abilities.

The fourth year of the School's programme is dedicated to internship activities, both in hospital and the community, with six months' experience in each field. This approach offers endless opportunities for practical experience in nutrition care of ambulatory patients who require special diets, food service management, and applied nutrition programmes.

The community nutrition programme is developed in Chimaltenango and places particular emphasis on the multidisciplinary team approach, which leads towards the solution of the community's nutritional problems. At a given demonstration-site, senior students from the School of Nutrition, together with final-year students from the University of San Carlos de Guatemala's Schools of Medicine, Dentistry, Social Work, and Veterinary Medicine, work jointly in the planning, implementation, and evaluation of specific programmes in surrounding rural villages. All of them are oriented to improve the health and nutritional status of the population. The same project involves promoting availability of foods, teaching better nutritional practices, and providing adequate care through supplementary feeding programmes, day nurseries, and patient care in general.

During the internship period, special research projects for practical application are planned accordingly in these different areas of experience and presented in thesis form, which is a requisite for graduation.

Upon completion of the curriculum, students are granted the degree of 'Licenciado'. This is equivalent to that of a university Bachelor of Science, with the added features of thesis preparation and internship as part of the academic requirements.

RESULTS

The School's first group graduated in 1969. Up to the present a total of 73 students have graduated and 27 are nearing completion of their thesis work. Of the total group, 36 are already working in applied nutrition with the Ministries of Health of the Central American countries, 17 work in institutional dietetics, and 17 in educational programmes.

DISCUSSION

While progress of the programme could be measured in terms of the number of graduates, we must emphasize that its implications are indeed overwhelming.

Firstly, the School acts as a laboratory school for the rest of Latin America. In fact, in 1966 its curriculum served as the basis of discussion at the First Meeting of Directors of Schools of Nutrition in Caracas, Venezuela. Gradually, after this meeting took place, the curriculum of most of the other Latin American Schools has been adapted to the recommendations expressed on that occasion.

Secondly, the multiplication effect will soon render fruitful results. In two of the area countries efforts are being made to establish a national school of nutrition to function under the leadership of our graduates.

Thirdly, the research work carried out by the students is widening knowledge of the nutrition problems of the area, especially of those related to nutrition education and other applied fields.

In our opinion, future plans for the School should include:

(1) a follow-up study of the graduates' experiences so as to discover emerging goals or new approaches to the formation of human resources in nutrition; and

(2) continuing education programmes for those graduates already involved in nutrition activities.

24 Nutrition education in catering studies in the UK

CONOR REILLY

INTRODUCTION

To most professional nutritionists and food scientists it would appear self-evident that nutrition should find a place in hotel and catering studies. However, the assumption is challenged not only by the existence of some catering educational programmes devoid of all nutrition, but also by the results of a survey carried out by the Hotel, Catering, and Institutional Management Association (HCIMA 1977). In addition, practical difficulties as well as student opposition frequently support the contrary view.

Nevertheless, courses in catering have almost invariably included 'science' in the syllabus, and many hotel managers and others in the catering industry have been exposed to it in their professional training. The results have not invariably been happy and it cannot be said that the science of nutrition plays much part in the professional life of all hotel managers today.

This case-study describes an attempt to remedy faults in teaching which have led not to antagonism but rather to negative attitudes towards food science and nutrition.

THE PROBLEM

In 1973 at the Oxford Polytechnic some 250 students were taking Higher National Diplomas in Hotel, Catering, and Institutional Management. The syllabus for this three-year course followed guidelines laid down by a joint committee representing industry, the Ministry of Education, and professional organizations. Four out of the total weekly timetable of twenty-eight hours were devoted to applied science. The course could equally well have been followed by students taking any of the other diploma courses available in the Polytechnic and could have been taught by service teachers with no specialist interest in catering.

Experience showed that after the Foundation Science Programme it was difficult to win back the interest of catering students to such topics as nutrition and hygiene.

With backing from Ministry of Education inspectors and Polytechnic administrators, we introduced an interim modified programme in which we were able to dispense largely with outside service teaching and teach science within the context of catering.

Some improvement of student attitudes was quickly observed. We took advantage of the situation to prepare for long-term changes. As non-catering scientists we, like the students, had to learn also about the place science could play in vocational studies. With help from several of the professional caterers in the department we devised a new syllabus which was introduced in 1975.

AIM

Our aim was not to make food scientists out of our students, but rather to help them appreciate the place of science in catering; we wanted to broaden their horizons and help them arrive at a position where they could make informed judgements about science and the new technologies which were making impact on the traditional crafts and expertise of the caterer.

THE PROGRAMME

We recognized that many of our students were not primarily interested in science; many of them had chosen catering because they had not done well at science in school, if they had done any at all. Moreover, among those who had science there was a very wide range of attainment. Rather than give them all a possibly, for some, boring foundation course, we adopted a 'Self-Learn Science Scheme' (Milson 1974). This was suitable for both beginners and advanced students and allowed them all to reach a comparable starting-point for further studies, but at their own pace. About one hour a week was given to it. It was felt that an attempt should be made to expose the catering students at the same time to hygiene, an area of applied science which we believed did not demand a science background and which, because of its novelty, could not be considered boring. The course was deliberately practical, kitchen-centred, and illustrated the pertinence of science to professional catering.

On the basis of this initial exposure to applied science and utilizing the foundations laid in the Self-Learn Scheme, the second term was devoted to an 'Introduction to Food Science'. As far as possible illustrations came from catering, and liaison with other staff allowed much pertinent application to actual problems. In Terms 3 and 4 Human Biology, Nutrition, and Dietetics were introduced, again with a close connection to practical catering. This was a taught programme, but once more the differing backgrounds of students caused problems and this section is now being modified to include a Biology Self-Learn Scheme.

RESULTS

It is hard to say at this stage what has been the result, long-term, of the new syllabus. Student reaction has been good, with less obvious reluctance to participate. For staff, teaching has been easier and more rewarding. Perhaps the best tribute is that twenty of the third year students have expressed an interest in the applied science option in nutrition. This is in marked contrast to previous years when we had only a handful of takers.

PROPOSALS FOR THE FUTURE

We do not believe we have finally solved the problem of making science an acceptable and fruitful part, as it should be, of catering studies, but we have at least made it appear more pertinent to the professional education of hotel, catering, and institutional managers. By accepting the fact that science cannot be taught as an extra, but must be integrated and be seen by students and all staff to be a valid part of catering, we seem to have made some progress. But a lot remains to be done. We would like to progress further, with close integration of science in professional training. We would like to see a programme in which there was not division, at least on timetable and syllabus, between, for example, kitchen management and hygiene and, if the same member of staff could not actually teach both, then the closest liaison and time-sharing should exist between them. Could not larder studies and food commodities be studied along with aspects of food chemistry? And where better than in menu-planning could nutrition and dietetics be found? We have a lot more to do in these areas following the example of such excellent texts as McWilliams (1974) and Smith and Minor's *Food service science* (1974). More could also be made of experimental cookery as a training in the application of the scientific method to food prep-aration, rather than as a sort of advanced cookery skills as it is in many catering courses. Here Griswold (1970) is a good guide.

REFERENCES

Griswold, R.M. (1970). *The experimental study of foods*. Constable, London.
HCIMA (1977). *The profile of professional management*. Hotel, Catering and Institutional Management Association, London.
McWilliams, M. (1974). *Food fundamentals* (2nd edn.) J. Wiley, New York.
Milson, A. (1974). *Applied science, chemistry and physics*. Sheffield Polytechnic, Department of Hotel and Institutional Management.
Smith, L.L.E. and Minor, L.J. (1974). *Food service science*. Avi, Westport, Conn.

25 Pilot scheme on nutrition education at the primary stage in India

G. GURU

BACKGROUND SETTING

There is a blending of ecological, religious, and socio-economic factors in the evolution of the pattern of diet among different categories of the population of India. The majority of the population are vegetarian, with the availability of milk acting as a limiting factor in the development of vegetarianism. Milk is preferred by most, when available. Flesh food (except beef) would be acceptable to the non-vegetarian population if economically available (especially fish, mutton, and chicken). Dietic variation centres round the locally available principal staples which, in order of importance, are rice, wheat, and different kinds of millet. Pulses enter as a regular component in the diet when money allows, especially in the north.

Of the protein consumed by an average Indian, 60 per cent comes from cereals and 26 per cent from pulses and nuts. Only a small portion is supplied from animal sources. Thus an imbalance in essential amino acids occurs, especially methionine, lysine, and trytophan. It is estimated (1968) that there is a protein gap of 3.65 million tons per year.

Fifty-eight grams of vegetables, including starchy roots, are available per capita per day in India, against the requirement of 284 g (114 g leafy vegetables, 85 g root vegetables, and 85 g other vegetables).

This deficit is reflected in the nutritional and health status of the country. The total caloric intake is less than that required for healthy living. The diet includes more carbohydrates and is short of animal proteins and fats. About 60 per cent of the population suffer from protein deficiency. Malnutrition is widely prevalent among the vulnerable sections of the population, namely, children and expecting and lactating mothers. Population below the age of 11 years constitutes 42 per cent of the Indian population, and nearly 75 per cent of these are malnourished. The low level of food supplies is of great concern to the Government of India.

The reasons are not only poverty and non-availability of food, but also to a large extent ignorance of nutritional facts and nutritionally undesirable practices and beliefs about food.

THE IMPORTANCE OF NUTRITION EDUCATION AT THE PRIMARY STAGE

Since education is the best platform to help eradicate such problems, a nutrition education programme which reaches the vulnerable section of the population in the quickest possible time in the existing situation with the means available at hand has become a vital necessity.

At present there are 60 million children in the primary stage. They constitute 71 per cent of the school population and 80 per cent of the population of the 6-10 age-group. The primary school period is the most impressionable one in the life of an individual and, as such, desirable nutritional habits can be easily inculcated at this stage. The introduction of nutrition education at the primary stage is therefore crucial in launching any dynamic national nutrition programme. In this way, a majority of the vulnerable section lf the population will be reached—not only 60 million children and 1.5 million teachers, but also parents through child-parent and teacher-parent interaction.

PILOT SCHEME

To achieve the above goal, the first step has been taken by launching the pilot scheme on nutrition, health education, and environmental sanitation in the primary stage, which is sponsored by the Government of India through the National Council of Educational Research and Training (NCERT) and assisted by UNICEF under the Science Education Programme.

The scheme was virtually started at the three-day national conference in August 1975 at Coimbatore, in which the Honorary Directors of the Regional Centres and the members of the NCERT, UNICEF, and ICAR associated with the programme took part. The Conference worked out the general strategy and guidelines of implementation.

OBJECTIVES

The general objectives of the pilot scheme are as follows:

(1) to enable children and those who take care of them to understand that proper nutrition is essential for good health and normal physical and mental development;
(2) to educate them in the selection, preparation, and conservation of good-quality foods; and
(3) to develop desirable practices in food hygiene, and environmental sanitation.

The expected outcomes are:

(1) improved awareness and knowledge of nutrition, health, and environmental sanitation of the target group—children, teachers, and parents;

(2) changes in food habits;
(3) improvement of nutritional and health status in terms of height and weight and, when possible, the clinical picture through school health and inspection;
(4) increased food production through school- and kitchen gardens;
(5) improvement in school attendance; and
(6) reduction in mortality.

DESIGN

The scheme is purely experimental in nature and is expected to be completed in three years.

To take care of the diversity of conditions, food habits, etc. prevailing in different parts of the country, five regional centres—one each in the southern, eastern, western, northern, and central parts of the country—were established during 1975.

The locations of the centres are as follows:

Region	Location
Southern	Sri Avinashilingam Home Science College for Women Coimbatore, Tamil Nadu.
Eastern	Biharilal College of Home and Social Science Judges Court Road, Calcutta, West Bengal.
Western	Department of Food and Nutrition, Faculty of Home Science, M.S. University Baroda, Gujarat.
Northern	College of Home Science Punjab Agricultural University, Ludhiana, Punjab.
Central	State Institute of Science Education Jabalput, M.P.

To implement the scheme the Department of Education in Science and Mathematics of NCERT was made responsible for general planning, co-ordination, and overall evaluation at national level.

At the State level, the Department of Education is responsible for overall guidance, supervision, and all administrative arrangements and implementation strategy.

The specific tasks of each Regional Centre are:

(1) to prepare, test, and develop appropriate packages of instructional material on nutrition (as well as health and sanitation) suited to primary school stage, which should be easily integrated in the teaching–learning process without increasing the teaching load, cost, or time of pupils, teachers, and management;
(2) to prepare, test, and develop instructional material for training of teachers with the ultimate aim of bringing about the necessary change in teacher training centres;

(3) to help the teachers to understand and practise the techniques of integrating nutrition–health concepts in the different subjects in schools;

(4) to test and devise ways and means by which nutrition and health education can be concurrently imparted to out-of-school groups.

One rural district per state per centre would be the operational basis to implement the scheme. The first phase of experiment would be limited to 100–150 schools, preferably one block. In the second phase, the experiment would be extended to 400 more schools in the selected district. It was envisaged that the packages developed through the experiment would be subsequently introduced in more and more schools, as well as teacher-training schools, with the ultimate objective of covering the whole country.

PROGRESS

The curriculum guide on nutrition/health education and environmental sanitation in primary schools was developed in a workshop at Baroda in January 1976 (NCERT 1976) and included chapters on objectives, content and its organization, teaching strategy, evaluation, model text for students, teachers' activities and training programmes. It was developed to cater to the needs of the five Regional Centres by providing guidelines to (a) curriculum planners and evaluators, (b) the writing team in textual material and teachers' guide, (c) the teacher–educators and supervisors, and (d) classroom teachers. During the first year, the regional centres took their own time to establish all administrative and academic arrangements and form the working group. The working group was comprised in each case of a representative of the State Department of Education, the UNICEF Zone Officer, Field Advisers of NCERT and the regional centres to co-ordinate and guide the entire activities.

Out of the five centres, Coimbatore, having a crash programme, had the responsibility of introducing the scheme in 10 blocks of the district, involving 600 schools with 3000 teachers. The project has now been carried out in the following steps:

(1) incorporation of health and nutrition education in the existing curricula of elementary schools and related institutions;

(2) production, try-out of instructional material and teaching aids, reform and improvement of teacher education; and

(3) extension of educational services in the field of nutrition and health education to out-of-school groups.

Tasks accomplished include:

(1) one-month orientation course for the method masters of teacher training schools in Coimbatore;

(2) nutrition incorporated syllabus for the primary schools;

(3) an instructional manual on nutrition in Tamil, for the use of primary-school teachers;

(4) publication of audio-visual materials on the importance of nutrition and its relation to health;

(5) two-day seminar on nutrition education for the educational officers of Coimbatore District;

(6) a bench-mark survey was conducted in four Blocks from 3900 samples in order to know the food habits of the children and their parents; and

(7) training of 3461 primary-school teachers from ten selected blocks drawn from 660 schools.

The training programme was a great success. The attendance was 100 per cent. The teachers were very enthusiastic. They were eager to know more about nutrition-deficiency diseases, which are urgent everyday problems, and food and its importance.

The National Conference on the scheme was held from 23 to 27 June 1977 to review the progress of the work in all the centres and work out future guidelines and implementation strategy.

CONCLUSION

A short period is still left for the completion of the project. During this period revision of training packages and instructional materials, production of training packages for pre- and in-service training courses, and final evaluation of the scheme will be accomplished. However, the interim report suggests that fulfilment of objective (c) above will require a special programme.

REFERENCES

Choudhury, B. *Vegetables—their problems and prospects in India.* (Presidential address at the Section of Agricultural Sciences at the 61st Session of Indian Science Congress). Indian Science Congress Association, Calcutta.

Government of India (1976). *India, a reference annual 1976.* Ministry of Information and Broadcasting, New Delhi.

NCERT (1975). *Third all-India educational survey, some provisional statistics on school education.* NCERT, New Delhi.

NCERT (1976). *The curriculum guide on nutrition/health education and environmental sanitation in primary schools.* NCERT, New Delhi.

NCERT (1977). *Third all-India educational survey (School Education), National Tables, Volume I, Main Findings.* Survey and Data Processing Unit, NCERT, New Delhi, 1977.

NCERT. *Progress reports from regional centres on nutrition education.* (Office documents). NCERT, New Delhi.

Randhawa and Jain (1958). *Agriculture and animal husbandry.* Indian Council of Agricultural Research, New Delhi.

UNESCO (1975). *Teachers' study guide on the biology of human populations.* UNESCO Press, Paris.

UNICEF (1975). *Pilot scheme on nutrition/health education and environmental sanitation in the primary stage.* SEP Project I MPO. UNICEF, New Delhi.

White, R.O. (1974). *Rural nutrition in monsoon Asia.* University Press, Kuala Lumpur.

26 A nutrition education curriculum for Grade 9 students

MARLENE HAMILTON

PLAN OF ACTION

Agency: UNESCO/School of Education, University of the West Indies, Jamaica. Time: October 1976 to June 1977.

BACKGROUND OF THE PROBLEM

Nature of the problem

Available statistics reveal a serious picture of malnutrition in Jamaica. In 1965, for example, a total of 689 persons died from nutritional deficiency; in 1969 the number was 552, and in 1970, 534 deaths were recorded. The following details may also be added.

1. The 534 deaths from malnutrition in 1970 represented (from 121 categories of fatal illnesses reported) the seventh largest category numerically.

2. Of these 534 fatalities 471 (253 males and 218 females) were under the age of 5 years (i.e. 0.2 per cent of the island's population under the age of 5, and 18 per cent of all deaths recorded for this age group).

3. There were a further 751 deaths reported in 1970 for the under-five group, which arose indirectly as a result of malnutrition (excluding still-births from malnutrition). When this number of fatalities is totalled with that attributed directly to malnutrition (i.e. 471) 40.2 per cent of all deaths is accounted for in the relevant age-group.

The nutritional problems identified in 1973 by a committee working on a food and nutrition policy for Jamaica included the following.

1. About one-fifth (approximately 50 000) of the children under 4 years of age were significantly underweight for their age.

2. Some 3 per cent of the island's two-year-olds were severely malnourished and required urgent treatment.

3. The mortality rate among children in the age range 1 to 4 years was 4.5 per thousand.

4. About 45 per cent of the pregnant and lactating mothers were anaemic, thus causing complications for the infants.

5. Many children were attending school without adequate breakfast.

6. Weights and heights of schoolchildren of low-income families were significantly lower than those from middle- and upper-class families.

7. Some 30 per cent of pre-school, and an undetermined number of school-age children, did not receive sufficient energy and protein food.

8. Agricultural workers, during periods of heavy labour, lost weight—a fact which was said to indicate a deficient energy intake. These problems were largely attributed to the stage of the island's food supply, certain characteristics of this being as follows:

(a) in the aggregate, energy-food supplies available in Jamaica in 1972 were 30 per cent above the quantity recommended for the island, while proteins were 70 per cent above;

(b) for low-income groups, the most important sources of energy are sugar, flour, and rice, and of protein, flour, rice, and bread; and

(c) low-income families depend on imported salt fish as an important source of protein, rather than on locally produced eggs and chickens.

While the above-mentioned data may be correct for Jamaica in general it must be realized that patterns of food consumption vary in different parts of the island, these being determined by:

1. *Availability of food.* In the past more emphasis was placed on the production of crops for export than on domestic food crops; only 6 per cent of all farm lands is devoted to domestic crops, and a large proportion of arable land is not being cultivated. The efficiency of local food-production is relatively low, and owing to poor storage there is a high wastage of farm products. The low earning-power of many families (e.g. very large families with small incomes) restrict their dietary intake.

2. *Food prices and income.* Owing to domestic problems (and also problems of the world market) the price of food has increased considerably, when compared with incomes. In 1972 40 per cent of Jamaica's employed labour-force earned less than $520 a year; 42 per cent earned less than $1560, and about 25 per cent of the adult population was unemployed. Owing to high food prices and low wages many did not have enough to eat.

3. *Knowledge, attitudes, and beliefs.* Some people are underfed because of:
(a) a lack of knowledge of the nutritional value of foods; and
(b) religious or cultural beliefs, which result in taboos being placed on some foods. In addition, consumers are sometimes misguided by advertisements, while others judge the nutritional value of foods in accordance with cost.

The above discussion does not present a favourable picture. While factors such as improved medical care, greater food production, and other relevant interventions will undoubtedly bring about a reduction of these problems, in order than any improvement may be maintained, education in nutrition remains essential.

THE DESIGN FOR IMPLEMENTATION OF THE PROJECT

The sample

Limitations of time and shortage of suitably skilled personnel have

made it necessary to confine the project to one educational level—
the New Secondary School—and to one specific grade—Grade 9.
This selection has been justified because of the following considerations:

1. New Secondary education in Jamaica initially spanned three years,
    hence Grade 9 was the terminal grade.

2. In any experimental work, one must as far as possible control the inter-
    ference of certain variables. For this reason, one would not wish to
    sample pupils entering secondary school for the first time (Grade 7),
    since they would naturally be facing a period of adjustment; the use of
    more advanced grades should better serve the purposes of the project.

3. Grade-9 pupils would currently be in their third year of secondary
    training, by which time we believe they would be ready to grapple with
    scientific concepts. Since much of nutrition education is achieved through
    science teaching, Grade-9 pupils should have had the prerequisites for a
    fuller appreciation of the material to be taught.

Although Jamaica is a small country, its environmental factors vary
considerably. Socio-economic conditions, agricultural methods,
nutritional habits, educational exposure, health care, etc., admit of
extremes of differences as between one place and another. Thus the
project is being implemented in two New Secondary Schools in
contrasting environments, both outside the Kingston conurbation
where schools tend to be overworked by local researchers. These two
schools are identified as:

School A (Seaforth New Secondary School)—located in the parish
of St. Thomas, almost in the middle of a sugar-cane plantation.

School B (Ocho Rios New Secondary School)—located on the
north coast in the midst of the tourist centre of Jamaica. Compared with School A, this school is in a prosperous environment.

Design

The UNESCO Guide (Griffin and Light 1975) suggests three alternative ways of curriculum structure.

1. The rational–empirical design, whereby teachers concern themselves
    with 'what behaviours are desired of students after a period of instruction,
    the activities being chosen because they can be assured to produce these
    behaviours'.

2. The 'engagements curriculum' design, which calls for greater participation
    on the part of students in the curriculum-making process. 'Great faith is
    placed upon the contact the students make with what is provided in the
    school, home and community environment,' and this is 'dependent
    upon belief and value systems'.

3. The 'emergent curriculum' design. Here, the pupil is the central factor and must decide what he wants to know and when he wants to learn it.

After discussions with local resource personnel, the decision has been taken to orient the project according to the 'engagements' model. It was felt that use of the engagements model should provide wide scope for activities which would be most meaningful and relevant to the students, necessitating as it does active participation by students in the curriculum-making process. It was also felt that this model applied in widely contrasting areas of Jamaica should make for interesting differences regarding material selected for inclusion by the pupils. (On this point, a small pilot survey showed pupils at School A to be interested in the food requirements of manual workers, such as cane cutters, while at School B, interest centred around sedentary workers, such as secretaries and hotel receptionists. Further, nutritional illnesses of interest at School A ranked high on their list of priorities, while at School B this was not the case.)

Other aspects identified for structuring a curriculum according to the engagements design seemed feasible for the purpose of this project.

1. The teachers involved could see to it that the complexity of content and method of presentation was suitable to Grade-9 students.

2. No doubt (as indicated from the pilot survey) activities would be selected by students on the basis of the inherent integrity of the activities, their value in the particular culture (or sub-culture), and their use in providing opportunities for students to react to concepts about the most valued goods and services of the society. Hence the students' thinking should become engaged with valued skills, knowledge, and ideas.

Implementation procedures

It has already been pointed out that some training in nutrition is offered in different subject areas. It is therefore felt that the implementation of the project within such subject areas might yield interesting results. Hence, plans are to introduce the project in the following way:

At School A: through general science, home economics, and agriculture.

At School B: through general science and home economics (no agriculture is offered at this school).

The top-stream Grade-9 pupils are to be involved, together with their regular teachers of the respective subject areas. Since these schools operate a shift system, in each instance every experimental group will be matched with a control group taught according to the regular curriculum of the Ministry of Education. The project co-ordinator will provide overall supervision, and inputs are promised from the following resource personnel:

Education Officers of the Ministry of Education, Jamaica, responsible for general science, home economics, and agriculture at the secondary level. These persons will provide help in structuring the curriculum with a specific slant towards their respective curriculum areas.

An Extension Officer of the Ministry of Agriculture and Lands, who has agreed to visit both schools and hold sessions with the students participating in the project.

A Research Officer (in the area of nutrition) at the Scientific Research Council, who has agreed to visit both schools and participate as a resource person.

Staff at the University of the West Indies (School of Education, Caribbean Food and Nutrition Institute, Science Centre, Social and Preventive Medicine), who have agreed to offer guidance in the making of lesson plans.

Proposed method of evaluation

1. For each group (control and experimental) the following basic information will be ascertained:
   (a) age of students;
   (b) mental ability score (determined by a standardized local test developed by Professor L.H.E. Reid of the University of the West Indies);
   (c) reading comprehension level (determined by local test developed by Irwin of the University of the West Indies);
   (d) the socio-economic status of the students; and
   (e) the ratio of boys to girls.
   While (d) and (e) will mainly be of use for descriptive purposes, it is planned that (a) to (c) will be treated statistically to establish relative homogeneity of the sample.

2. An achievement test in nutrition (multiple-choice items) is to be constructed and administered to students prior to the teaching of any material. The same test will be administered at the end to determine any incremental gain (pre-test/post-test design).

3. The most important instrument (for the purpose of this project) will be that which calls for evaluation of the lessons by both students and their teachers. This will be structured according to UNESCO's guidelines, tapping areas of specific interest to the pupil's valuable aspects of the project, and evidence of continued interest.

4. Observations of lessons in progress will be made, possibly with the help of the Flander's Interaction Schedule.

5. An impressionistic evaluation by four experienced educators, including two who are scientists and were not involved in running the programme. These persons would visit the classrooms, inspect the instructional materials and examine the course and the teaching. The visits would be made on three occasions at intervals of at least a month.

Goals of the proposed project

The interdisciplinary nature of nutrition in our estimation warrants implementation of this project as planned—via the subject areas of general science, home economics, and agriculture. The inclusion of students in the decision-making process—having them decide which aspects they want to learn, adopting these and using local illustrations —should make for greater effort on their part.

However, the aim is not only to attain in students an understanding of the basic principles of nutrition, but also to encourage appreciation of its importance to themselves and to the community as a whole. Hopefully, if the seed of awareness is firmly implanted in these students, there will be cause to expect some of its positive effects to filter beyond the limits of the classroom in time. Generally speaking, the project should test certain assumptions and insights about curriculum and methods in the area of nutrition.

Limitations

Certain limitations have already been recognized—namely the time factor involved and the shortage of suitably skilled personnel. As regards time, only one term (10 weeks) can be allowed. Adjustments to the curriculum can therefore be barely minimal. The limitation of time has made it impossible for attitudinal changes in students to be identified, and this is regrettable, since one of the main aims of nutrition educational programmes is to foster favourable attitudes in participants.

One also recognizes a local phenomenon in the inconsistent attendance of Jamaican students at school (especially in rural areas), as well as the fact that mid-term examinations dictate a break in the sequencing of the project at School A. Nonetheless, the project is being implemented as planned in both schools and, provided the evaluation techniques reflect awareness of the stated limitations, reasonably reliable results will be forthcoming.*

REFERENCES

Griffin, G.A. and Light, L. (1975). *Nutrition education curricula: relevance, design, and the problem of change.* UNESCO.

*This project has now been completed and a report will be published as a UNESCO document in the near future.

27 Non-governmental organizations — link schemes: the experience at the University of Ife

G.R. HOWAT

One method by which nutrition education at University level has been advanced in the developing countries is by the use of 'link schemes'. In these schemes a well-established university, usually in one of the industrialized countries, establishes a formal link with another university or other institution of higher learning. Although these links are for mutual help, it is understood that it is that part of the link in the developing country which is the greater beneficiary.

The necessary funding of the link schemes is borne by one or other of the large international organizations or charitable foundations. In the case of the UK funding is done by the Inter-University Council which has been established through the Overseas Development Ministry of the British Government.

In 1969 UNESCO published a document entitled, *Bilateral links in science and technology*. This was the result of a study of many link schemes which were then in existence between educational and research institutions in Europe and North America and similar institutions in the developing world. It gave details of the subject fields concerned and sometimes of the extent of financial involvement of the link. Most, but not all, of the links were between universities.

More recently (in 1975) the Inter-University Council published a document entitled, *Co-operation through links*, which is essentially the report of a working party of the Council on the operation of the very many links which the Council, since 1965, has sponsored between Universities in the United Kingdom and similar institutions in other countries in the Commonwealth. These links cover a wide range of disciplines and have included some in which nutrition education is involved.

One of the best known of these is the link between the Department of Food Science at the University of Reading and the Department of Food Science and Technology at the University of Ife, Nigeria. It was set up early in 1971 when the Department at the University of Ife was established and its main purpose was to facilitate the development of that Department.

From the viewpoint of those at Ife the link made special pro-vision, including the necessary finance where necessary, for the following:

(1) contact with the long-established and highly regarded Department of Food Science at Reading on all matters relating to the new Department.

(2) a Head of Department at Ife for a period of five years on official leave from the University of Reading;

(3) visits by the staff at Ife to the University of Reading and other Uni-versities in the United Kingdom and also to research centres for dis-cussion on food and nutrition matters;

(4) visits by staff at Reading to Ife as external examiners, visiting lecturers, and speakers at seminars on specialist topics, e.g. oils and fats technology and sensory evaluation of foods;

(5) visits by staff at Ife to scientific conferences in the UK and elsewhere on food and nutrition matters; and

(6) periods of study for higher degrees for staff and post-graduate students at Reading or elsewhere in the UK.

There is no doubt that the Department at Ife benefited from the link to a greater extent than the Department at Reading. Nevertheless the link provided the staff at Reading with the stimulus of seeing at first hand the challenge of teaching food and nutrition science in a community where the social framework and cultural background were different from those in Western Europe. It also gave them an insight—sometimes by being involved in the research problems of the staff at Ife—into the difficulties which arise in nutritional and other matters in one of the developing countries.

One aspect of the work on nutrition education—in addition to the formal nutrition courses which were an integral part of the under-graduate—can best be described as extension work. Two methods were established.

The first was collaboration with staff in the Departments of Home Economics in the teacher training colleges. We found that the staff in these Departments were most anxious to pass on to their students up-to-date information on nutrition matters. Members of the staff of the Department at Ife visited the colleges and gave lectures on appropriate nutrition topics. Members of staff of the colleges to-gether with their students paid return visits to Ife and saw the work which was going on there.

The second method was the publication of a quarterly journal, *Nigeria Nutrition Newsletter*. Nigeria is short on locally produced glossy magazines for women readers such as the women's weeklies and monthlies which are so popular in Europe and North America and which often give useful articles on nutrition and diet specially oriented towards the young mothers. So we decided to produce our own quarterly publication aimed at the general reader, both male and female.

Since the publication could not be described as academic we decided not to approach the University for funds. Instead we approached a few of the large food-processing companies in Nigeria. They responded well—although the Newsletter carries no advertising matter—and the first four issues were largely financed by them.

In its general layout and style the Newsletter owes much to a similar publication, *Cajanus*, published by the Carribean Food and Nutrition Institute in Jamaica, and so far the response to it by the general public has been good. As would be expected from what has been said about the teacher training colleges they are heavy subscribers and through them we hope that in due time so also will the larger schools.

In addition to link schemes, a wide variety of agencies are offering nutrition education to those with whom they are in contact. These agencies are mainly registered charitable foundations and bodies such as the Christian Missions and Churches.

The scope of the nutrition education programmes so presented varies widely both in scope and character. And, it must be added, in technical quality. Very often it is only when clinical systems of malnutrition exist that advice on nutritional matters is given. Little attention appears to be given to nutrition education to persons who are, or at least appear to be, in good health. It is clear that there is a need for nutrition education to be given as part of the normal educational programmes in schools and also for the subject to be raised at community groups in the same way as other subjects are discussed.

REFERENCES

Inter-University Council (1975). *Co-operation through links.*
UNESCO (1969). *Bilateral links in science and technology.* UNESCO.

Section IV
Review of the conference

At a conference dealing with nutrition education it was to be expected that both nutritionists and educationists would be well represented. Such was the case, and although both groups were competent in their disciplines and articulate in their own fields it quickly became apparent that developments in nutrition education required a fully co-operative approach. The nutritionists required the skills of the educators for effective communication while the educationists needed to acquire—or at least have supplied to them—all manner of nutritional background information.

Although this was the first major international conference to deal with the subject it was clearly recognized that nutrition education is far from being a new activity. Indeed, especially in the non-formal educational sphere, nutrition education has been taking place in a pragmatic manner for many centuries in what are now the industrialized countries as well as in the present developing countries. Nevertheless the need for a more formal approach is well recognized in view of the widespread ignorance—or possibly disregard for existing knowledge—in dietary matters.

The field of formal education is of more recent origin but is already well-established at least in so far as girls and women students are concerned. In secondary schools for many years there have been departments of home economics (formerly called departments of domestic science) which had a recognized place for nutritional matters in their curricula. Unfortunately no similar information on nutritional matters was passed on to boys and young men, except sometimes through biology classes.

In recent years the establishment of departments of food science at some universities and other institutions of higher learning has provided better facilities for nutrition education to both young men and women. Nevertheless it is still true that most boys and young men lack formal nutritional education. This was a matter on which concern was expressed in discussion groups.

Even where nutrition education was given there appears to be no really satisfactory method so far of evaluating its effectiveness in influencing dietary behaviour. Nor is there adequate information available on what type of educational approach is most likely to have lasting results on the behaviour of the different population groups.

Both these points were noted as matters for concern in papers presented and in subsequent discussion.

It was considered generally that formal nutrition education (though not under that name!) could usefully start at the primary stage of school education. It was noted that even before that time there would be—in some societies at least—some non-formal education between the young child and the mother in which the child will have been informed of the 'goodness' of some foods and the need to consume them.

Some of the specialists in the field of primary education expressed the view that even in primary school an awareness should be created of the existence of the main types of food, that their coexistence constitutes nutritional balance, and that they are generally not interchangeable.

In secondary school, as a broader infrastructure of general knowledge develops, these concepts would be extended so that the word 'food' could be expressed, when appropriate, as 'nourishment'. From such a realization it was believed that the general principle could be established in the minds of young people that the right kind of food in the right quantity was an integral part of full bodily health.

The desirability of involving parents, as far as possible, in such education in the home situation was recognized but there was uncertainty how this could be done when, as sometimes was the case, the parents also were seriously deficient in nutritional knowledge.

The proposal was that at these schools where a midday meal is served teachers could explain why different items were normally incorporated in the meal. This proposal implied that the teachers themselves had adequate knowledge of the subject, a basis that could not always be relied on. Another proposal which received backing in discussion groups was that nutrition education in schools should include instruction on the relationship between the practice of sanitary habits in the storing, preparation, and cooking of food and the incidence of outbreaks of food poisoning, and also instruction on the recognition of food spoilage in common foods and its potential health hazards.

The position of the universities and other institutions of university rank was also closely considered in relation to nutrition education. Both in formal papers and in discussion groups special attention was given to the training of students who would in turn become nutritionists and nutrition educators. There was wide acceptance that in these institutions of higher learning a need existed for some structural framework, either as a department or some other separate teaching unit, which would provide much of the necessary basic training and also help to identify in the minds of others the principle that nutrition is a basic academic discipline.

At this level two special areas of study in nutrition were identified. The first was nutrition education in relation to medicine and to the health sciences generally. The second was nutrition in relation to food science and agriculture. As far as the first area was concerned it was generally accepted that a good case could be presented for establishing a department of human nutrition in any new medical faculty. This should be used, among other things, for the instruction of medical students in nutritional matters and also it should provide related courses for paramedical staff such as nurses, pharmacists, dieticians, and so on. In the second area there was a similar need for instruction in nutritional matters to be given to students reading for a degree in agriculture. Some courses in agriculture already included instruction in animal nutrition and it was clearly necessary for human nutrition to be included. Here also there was a need for a recognized centre, either as a full department or some other separate teaching unit, where nutrition education was provided.

It was in the field of non-formal education that there was very much discussion. In part this sprang from the special needs of the developing countries, many of which had urgent nutrition problems to solve. It was recognized that much non-formal nutrition education needed to be directed towards an adult audience in whom there were well-established dietary prejudices which could in some cases result in nutritional deficiences. It was therefore stressed that non-formal nutrition education must be carried out within a framework of intimate knowledge of the local social–political–economic situation. Without such knowledge there was a serious chance that non-formal nutrition education would lack the necessary relevance to enable it to be effective in its purpose.

One example of this was the importance of a nutritional message being transmitted by a high ranking person in the society concerned. He would be expected also to show by his example that he was practising the particular aspect of nutritional policy which he was transmitting to his audience. This was specially true in traditionally hierarchical societies.

One point believed to be important by some workers in the nutritional field in developing countries was the need for an integrated programme of nutrition education at all levels. This would mean that the timing of a national or regional campaign in non-formal education, e.g. by radio or TV, would coincide with formal instruction being given in schools at all levels. Co-ordination between different government departments was therefore necessary.

Special mention needs to be made of the discussions which centred round the potential contribution of the Paulo Freire method for education among illiterate adults. This method was conceived in north-east Brazil in the early 1960s and embodies a philosophy of education that aims at self-reliance and personality growth through the production of a critical consciousness on all environmental matters. 'Conscientization' is the word developed by Freire to express this critical awareness. The method involves the development of two-way communication between teachers and students regarding the subjects under study. Both teacher and students are considered to be learning.

Many of those who took part in the discussions and who had experience in the Freire method believed that it could have important applications among illiterate adults. These applications would include attitudes to kinds of food (especially taboos, myths, and preferences), eating habits, (meal times, social customs, division of food within families) and acceptance of studies on nutritional status (anthropo-metric indicators and observance of clinical symptoms). It was also believed by some members that the provision of time for open discussion on the Freire principle would be valuable when future conferences involving non-formal education of illiterate adults were under review.

Index